Speechreading

A Way to Improve Understanding
Second Edition, Revised

Harriet Kaplan

Scott J. Bally

Carol Garretson

Clerc Books

Gallaudet University Press, Washington, D.C.

Clerc Books
An imprint of Gallaudet University Press
Washington, DC 20002

Library of Congress Cataloging-in-Publication Data

Kaplan, Harriet.
    Speechreading: a way to improve understanding.

    Biography: p.
    Includes index.
    1.   Lipreading. 2. Lipreading—Study and teaching.
1. Bally, Scott J., 1945-   .II. Garretson, Carol, 1926-   .III. Title.
HV2487.K37   1987   371.91′27   87-7599
ISBN 0-930323-32-7

∞   The paper used in this publication mets the minimum requirements of American National
    Standards of Information Sciences—Permanence of Paper for Printed Library Materials, ANSI
    Z39.48-198

Contents

Chapters 1-4 and 6 are by Harriet Kaplan, Ph.D., Assistant Professor, Department of Audiology, Gallaudet University, Washington, D.C.

Chapter 5 and the introduction to chapter 7 are by Scott J. Bally, M.A., Clinical Supervisor, Department of Audiology at Gallaudet University.

The speechreading exercises in chapter 7 were organized and edited by Carol Garretson, M.A., former Assistant Professor, Department of Communication Arts at Gallaudet University.

Preface

According to estimates, there are approximately 20 million children and adults in the United States with some degree of hearing impairment (Chalfant & Sheffelin, 1969).* Habilitative/rehabilitative considerations are of primary concern for these people. Speechreading is an important part of habilitation or rehabilitation because all hearing-impaired individuals use this skill to some extent. Although speechreading has been taught in various ways for many years, only a few books are available explaining its many aspects. These books are texts written for the professional or professional-in-training and are oriented toward theory and research rather than the practical needs of the hearing-impaired person. There are also consumer-oriented books consisting only of speechreading exercises but no consumer-oriented text on the nature of speechreading itself.

The goal of *Speechreading: A Way to Improve Understanding* is to present the nature and process of speechreading and its benefits and limitations. The book was designed as a source of information for hearing-impaired adults of all ages and degrees of hearing loss, their families and friends, and parents of hearing-impaired children. It is hoped the book will clarify commonly held misconceptions and enable hearing-impaired people to use speechreading wisely and well. It is also our hope that the book may aid professionals and professionals-in-training in providing habilitative/rehabilitative services in classrooms and clinics.

Chapter 1 discusses principles of speechreading, its role in overall communication, how it can be used with residual hearing, and differences between good and poor speechreaders. Chapter 2 deals with the limitations of speechreading as they relate to the speaker, environment, and speechreader. It is important that these limitations be recognized so that compensatory strategies can be developed. In chapter 3 specific limitations relating to lack of visibility of some of the sounds of English are described. In addition, the issue of homopheneity, or the fact that some sounds look alike, is dealt with.

Chapter 4 discusses the desirability of assertive behavior as opposed to passive or aggressive behavior. Difficult communication situations and appropriate strategies to manage them are described. In chapter 5 programmed exercises illustrating the use of these communication strategies are presented. it is our hope that the material in these two chapters will help the reader cope with difficulties for which speechreading alone is insufficient.

---

*Chelfant, J. C., & Sheffelin, M. A. (1969). *Central processing dysfunction in children.* Bethesda, MD: U.S. Department of Health, Education & Welfare.

Chapter 6 discusses the problems inherent in the development of tests of speechreading skill. It also describes current methods of teaching speechreading. This chapter is designed to acquaint the reader with the ways in which speechreading is evaluated and taught.

The speechreading exercises in chapter 7 were designed by hearing-impaired students. They represent examples of the kinds of methodologies discussed in chapter 6 and are suitable for adolescents and adults.

Acknowledgments

The speechreading exercises in chapter 7, some of which have been edited to ensure format conformity, were developed by students in the Theories and Principles of Lipreading course at Gallaudet University. The authors wish to acknowledge all of the students who so graciously allowed their work to appear in this book, as well as Barbara Jarboe who contributed to the exercises on communication strategies. In addition, we wish to thank Jacqueline Sternberg of the Department of Audiology, Cynthia Vaughn of the Department of Communication Arts, and Pauline Peikoff of Alumni and Public Relations, Gallaudet University for their invaluable help in the preparation of this text.

Introduction

In order to understand speechreading as we know it, it is helpful to have some knowledge of its history. The history of speechreading is really part of the history of deaf education because it has always been one of the basic methods used to teach deaf individuals. Therefore, an overview of the history of deaf education, particularly oral-aural methodology, allows one to understand the development of the speechreading methods used today.

Early History of Deaf Education

Although deafness has been known since ancient times, until the sixteenth century prelingually deaf people were considered unteachable. In most societies they were classed with the mentally incompetent. The first known teacher of the prelingually deaf was a Spanish monk named Pedro Ponce de León who lived from 1520 to 1584. According to documents that he left, he was successful in teaching several deaf individuals, primarily using sign language (Deland, 1968).

Toward the end of the sixteenth century and the beginning of the seventeenth century, teachers in different parts of Europe began to develop methods to teach the deaf. Juan Martin Pablo Bonet in Spain introduced the idea that deaf children could be taught to speak by learning production of individual sounds through the senses of touch and vision. For speech understanding, he advocated the use of the manual alphabet rather than speech reading.

Around the same time, John Bulwer in England advocated use of a combination of sign language, speech, and "lip grammar" (speechreading). He regarded speechreading as a way of learning to speak rather than of understanding the speech of others.

Although these early deaf educators and others used both sign language and speechreading, they believed that speechreading was useful for speech production rather than speech understanding. They advocated the use of the manual alphabet and sign language for speech comprehension.

During the latter part of the seventeenth century and the early part of the eighteenth century, interest in speechreading spread to different parts of Europe. To a much greater extent, speechreading became recognized as a way of understanding language rather than a method of teaching speech.

Charles Michel de l'Epée, working in France, was one of the first to make education of the deaf available to the general public. Before 1755 whatever education existed for deaf children was restricted to the wealthy. de l'Epée opened a school for deaf children of Paris that was funded by the French government.

Originally, he included speech and speechreading in his curriculum but found that deaf children learned academic subjects faster with sign language. Since he needed to teach large numbers of children, he gave up the use of oral methods for a completely manual approach. After de l'Epée died, Abbé Sicard operated the school, continuing with the same methods. Manualism became the method of choice in France and spread to other parts of Europe and to America. Thomas Hopkins Gallaudet was greatly influenced by Sicard and another French teacher, Laurent Clerc.

At the same time de l'Epée and Sicard were developing the manual method in France, Samuel Heinicke was developing the oral method in Germany. Heinicke believed that clear thought was possible only through speech and that deaf people could be taught to understand speech by carefully watching a speaker's lips. He opened the first public school for the deaf in Germany, which was oral. After he died in 1790, his sons-in-law continued his work but chose to use the manual method. The oral method was not used again in Germany until it was reintroduced fifty years later by Friedrick Moritz Hill. Hill developed speech and language teaching to a high level, stressing that deaf children need to learn language naturally the way hearing children do by constant use rather than from grammar books. He also believed that speech must be the basis for teaching and communication. Many of the principles of oral deaf education as it is used today can be traced to Friedrich Hill. Despite his oral philosophy, he did not forbid the use of signing in the classroom.

Thomas Braidwood in England was a contemporary of both de l'Epée and Heinicke. He opened a private oral school which was continued by three generations of his family. A grandson started a small, semipublic school for deaf children in Virginia in 1813, but the school did not remain open long. The Braidwoods were very secretive about their ideas and refused to share them with others. Therefore, oralism with its emphasis on speechreading came to America from Germany rather than England.

Early Developments in America

The earliest methods of deaf education established in America were sign language and fingerspelling. At the beginning of the nineteenth century, Thomas Hopkins Gallaudet became interested in the education of deaf children and traveled to England to study the Braidwood methods. The Braidwoods, however, were concerned that Gallaudet would learn their procedures and then open a competing school in America. They offered to share their ideas only if he would accept a position in their school.

Gallaudet decided to study the sign and fingerspelling method of Sicard in France where he became friendly with a deaf teacher named Laurent Clerc. Clerc returned to America with Gallaudet and helped him start a school in

Hartford, Connecticut. This school became so successful that it received government funding. It was established as the American Asylum for the Deaf and is functioning today as the American School for the Deaf.

Following the opening of this first school in America, other states quickly started their own residential schools. These schools used sign language and fingerspelling, paying little attention to oral skills because of the current belief that deaf people were unable to speak.

Gradually some educators began to notice the success of oral methods in England and Germany. In 1867, John Clarke opened the first oral school in Northampton, Massachusetts. It was called the Clarke School for the Deaf and is the oldest of the oral schools in the United States. This was followed by the opening of an oral day school in Boston that, after 1873, became known as the Horace Mann School for the Deaf. Additional oral schools developed, and speechreading training was given increasing attention. Advocates of speech and speechreading became as well known as those using manual methods. By the latter half of the nineteenth century, the communication methods war started by de l'Epée, Heinicke, and Braidwood in Europe was in full swing in the United States.

In 1872 Alexander Graham Bell began a training class for teachers of the deaf in Boston. Because Bell was a strong advocate of oral deaf education, the teaching of lipreading was included in the curriculum. He believed that deaf children should be educated through speech and speechreading, preferably in day schools where they could have social contacts with hearing people and with their families. He established the Alexander Graham Bell Association for the Deaf, using prize money received from the invention of the telephone. This organization, located in Washington, D.C., serves as an advocacy group for oral deaf education, publishes materials for use by deaf and hard-of-hearing people, provides information about hearing impairment to the general public and professionals, and works with other organizations to lobby for the rights of the deaf.

During the second half of the nineteenth century a number of schools adopted what they called the simultaneous or combined method. The idea was to use the best of both oral and manual methodologies. In 1864 Gallaudet College, the only liberal arts college for the deaf in the world, was founded using the simultaneous communication method. The official communication policy is that speech or lip movements are to be used together with sign language and fingerspelling in all classes.

The concept of simultaneous communication evolved into the broader concept of total communication. Total communication is a philosophy which states that a deaf child has the right to be educated using any communication methodology or cgmbination of methods that best meets his or her needs. Despite the popularity of this concept, the conflict between those advocating oral-aural methods and those advocating predominantly sign language is still strong.

Excellent discussions of the history of deaf education can be found in Deland (1968), Berger (1972), and Moores (1978).

Adult Speechreading Programs

Until the 1890s the teaching of speechreading was largely limited to children as part of oral deaf education. At that time, however, some schools began to allow adults to participate along with the children. Very quickly, many speechreading teachers began to focus their attention on hard-of-hearing adults, and as a result four speechreading methods developed. All of our present procedures have evolved from these speechreading systems.

Around the beginning of the twentieth century, leagues for the hard of hearing began to form. These groups became powerful social service agencies for the hearing impaired. Some of the leagues were founded by well-known speechreading teachers who, together with hearing-impaired graduates of speechreading programs, became the first members. The earliest league was the New York League for the Hard of Hearing, founded in 1910 by Edward Nitchie and others. To this day, speechreading training offered by the New York League takes many of its ideas from the Nitchie speechreading method. Some of the goals of this organization were and still are

1. to establish organizations for the hard of hearing in the community;
2. to establish speechreading classes in the public schools for children and adults;
3. to encourage hearing testing of young children in the schools;
4. to encourage employers to hire deaf people;
5. to encourage hearing aid research;
6. to reach out to and provide services for isolated deaf people;
7. to cooperate in research into causes of deafness;
8. to encourage prevention of deafness;
9. to provide public education about deafness;
10. to function as an advocate for hearing-impaired people;
11. to provide hearing testing, hearing aid evaluations, speech, speechreading and listening training, and communication counseling.

The New York League served as a prototype for similar organizations throughout the country. In 1919 the groups united to form the American Association for the Hard of Hearing; it later changed its name to the National Association of Hearing and Speech Agencies (NAHSA) and still later to the National Association of Hearing and Speech Action. The community organizations that are members of NAHSA provide a great deal of professional service to hearing-impaired people, and NAHSA itself is affiliated with the American Speech-Language-Hearing Association.

Several formal speechreading methods were developed during the early years of the twentieth century. These methods are classified into *analytic* and *synthetic* approaches. The analytic approaches stress recognition of speech movements while deemphasizing use of contextual or situational clues. Synthetic methods emphasize use of language redundancy for speech understanding and minimize training in recognition of lip movements. Analytic methods focus on eye training and synthetic approaches emphasize mind training. Actually all speechreading methods have components of both eye and mind training but vary in their emphasis.

Early speechreading methods were largely analytic because speechreading was originally used as a method of improving speech production, a highly analytic skill. It was not until the 1870s that speechreading was considered to be a separate skill from articulation training. Therefore, emphasis was placed on teaching the student to analyze mouth positions as various sounds were produced. It was assumed that all speech sounds were at least partially visible. The student was expected to learn how each sound was produced. After the sound movement was learned, there was drill on repetition of syllables containing the sound or sounds. The next step was drill on words made from the syllables and finally on sentences containing those words. Meaningfulness of words or sentences was not considered important. In some of the earliest analytic methods, the sentences were almost nonsense.

The more modern speechreading methods are primarily synthetic, stressing understanding of meaningful, connected speech. Syllable drill is not used. Sentence material tends to focus on a single theme, often with one sentence logically following another. Some modern speechreading teachers do not use analytic methods at all; others use a slight amount of analytic training if needed for a particular student.

Of the four formal speechreading methods developed during the early twentieth century, none are either purely analytic or purely synthetic. Some, however, are more analytic than others. The Jena and Mueller-Walle are considered analytic while the Nitchie and Kinzie methods are considered synthetic. Every speechreading teacher today uses some combination of these procedures.

1. Principles of Speechreading

In this chapter the nature of speechreading, how it can help overall communication, and how it can be used with hearing will be discussed. Factors that make a person a good speechreader will also be discussed.

What Is Speechreading?

Many people are more familiar with an older term *lipreading*, which they interpret as the ability to recognize the different sounds of speech by observing movements of the lips, tongue, and jaw. The implication of this definition is that a skilled lipreader can interpret all speech movements and thereby substitute vision for hearing. Also implied is that this skill can be learned. This concept was probably fostered by early lipreading methods which stressed the recognition of speech movements.

Actually, skilled speechreaders depend on much more than the information available from the movements of the lips, tongue, and jaw. They interpret facial expressions, gestures, and body language and use clues available from the situation and what they know about the language. When the term *speechreading* was introduced, it was intended to include not only the more narrow concept of lipreading but also the other factors listed above. Therefore, a working definition of speechreading might be "the ability to understand a speaker's thoughts by watching the movements of the face and body and by using information provided by the situation and the language." Today, most people use the terms *lipreading* and *speechreading* interchangeably to mean use of all visual and situational information available.

Components of Speechreading

The vast majority of speechreading teachers do not emphasize recognition of individual sounds.

This skill is certainly important to speechreading, but the person who tries to recognize every sound as it is spoken will miss much of the information conveyed by the message. Therefore, sound recognition is not the component of speechreading that receives the most attention in training.

Gestures and Body Language

Gestures are mainly movements of the hands and arms, but they may also involve the head or other body parts. They are used in all cultures and may substitute for speech or supplement what the speaker says. Most gestures are used to supplement speech. An example is arm and hand movement to emphasize a point. Another example is glancing toward the people or objects being discussed. Following are some ways gestures can substitute for speech:

1. A nod of the head means "yes" or "I agree."

2. A beckoning movement of the hands or fingers can mean "come here."

On the hands of a skilled mime, gestures can almost be a complete language.

There have been a few studies on the contribution of natural gestures to speechreading. Berger, Martin, and Sataloff (1970) and Popelka and Berger (1971) demonstrated that understanding of speech improves significantly when appropriate gestures are used but deteriorates when the gestures are not appropriate.

Body language or body position is a form of gesture. This refers to how people sit, stand, or move their bodies. A person's mood can often be identified by body position or movement. A tired, unhappy, or bored person's shoulders may slump; a lowered head may indicate sadness or a dejected feeling. In contrast, a happy or enthusiastic person will probably stand upright with head held high.

Facial Expressions

Facial expressions, which are a common part of normal communication, can also supplement speechreading. A smiling face indicates happiness; raised eyebrows indicate questioning; a puzzled look suggests lack of understanding. The more expressive a speaker, the easier he or she is to understand. The more a speechreader can interpret facial expressions, the better he or she can understand.

Situational Clues

Situational clues include the place of the conversation and the roles of the people talking. The location can help you predict the kind of language used. For example, different things are said in a bank, a restaurant, the classroom, and a doctor's office. Furthermore, the speaker's role in a given situation affects what is said. In a restaurant, a waiter will not use the same language as your dinner companion. Situational clues help the speechreader predict the language used. You can predict what the waiter might say when he approaches your table because of his role in the situation. Since the possibilities are limited, it should not be difficult to resolve ambiguities seen on the lips.

Linguistic Factors

Language has a great deal of redundancy. This means there are many clues to understanding based on the structure of the language and many clues to correct interpretation of a spoken message occurring at the same time. Look at the sentence, I am the *teacher* in this class. You might understand the key word *teacher* by (*a*) the way it looks on the lips, (*b*) the way it sounds, or (*c*) what you could figure out from context (the sentence itself). All of that is redundancy. The more redundant a language, the less likely you are to make mistakes and the better you can function if some clues are missing such as a clearly heard message.

Language redundancy is provided by the rules of the language learned as children. The better you

know your language, the easier it is to speechread. Some rules used by most speechreaders/listeners follow.

1. There are a limited number of sounds in English, thirty-eight to be exact. All spoken messages must consist of only those sounds.

2. Sounds can be combined only in certain ways. In our language, /pr/ as in the word *pretty* is possible, but combinations such as /sr/ or /gt/ are not possible.

3. Parts of words (prefixes and suffixes) can be connected to main words only in certain ways. It is correct to say *coming* or *unhappy*, but not *ingcome* or *happyun*.

4. Words can be combined only in certain ways. In most English sentences, the subject comes first, then the verb, and then the object. For example, "He is going to the store" is correct, but "Going to the store he" is not acceptable.

5. The way in which words are spoken affects meaning. When people speak, they emphasize certain words to give meaning to what they say. They also vary intonation—the rise and fall of the voice in speaking. Where pauses occur in a sentence can also make a difference in meaning. Look at some examples.

> *Example A.* You're staying **home**.
> By emphasizing the last word and dropping the voice at the end of the sentence, the speaker tells the listener that she or he had better stay home. The message is even stronger if there is an angry look on the face and the hands are placed on the hips.

> *Example B.* **You're** staying home.
> Now the stress is on the word *you're*, meaning that *you* and not another person will stay home.

> *Example C.* You're staying **home**?
> This time the emphasis is on the last word but there is an upward tone of voice. There may also be a questioning look on the face. The meaning is quite different. Now we're asking a question.

Example D. I want the **milkman**.
With no pause between *milk* and *man*, the speaker is simply asking for the milkman. However, the meaning changes if a pause is inserted. The sentence—I want the milk, man—has a completely different meaning.

You might argue that these things are not really speechreading but are related to hearing and the use of information provided by gestures and facial expressions. Yet, this linguistic information may be considered part of the broader definition of speechreading: "The ability to understand a speaker's thoughts by watching the movements of the face and body and by using information provided by the situation and the language."

How do you use the redundancies of language to aid speechreading? Because what can be seen on the lips is limited, and because of the many ambiguities in the spoken message, you use the redundancies of language—situational clues, gestures, and facial expressions—to make good guesses. Knowledge of what the language structure permits allows you to fill in missing words or change words that do not make sense. For example,

Speaker says: Where *have* you been?

You speechread: Where *are* you been?

You think: *Are* does not make sense. It must be *have*.

While the speaker is talking, you may mentally replace words that seemed correct earlier in the conversation but now don't make sense because you have more information. For example,

You speechread: I saw her *mother* downtown yesterday.

You speechread later in the conversation: Her *mother* and father are living in Florida now.

You think: *Mother* couldn't have been right in the earlier sentence. Maybe the speaker said *brother*.

So, speechreading is a combination of what the eyes can see and the mind can correctly fill in. The work of the eyes is called the *analytic component* and work of the mind is called the *synthetic component*. Development of the analytic component is called *eye training* while development of the synthetic component is called *mind training*. Mind training is by far the most important part of speechreading. A good speechreader can take whatever is seen on the speaker's face, combine it with gestures, body language, facial expression, linguistic rules, situational clues, and whatever can be heard and make some sense of it.

Relationship to Hearing

The greater the hearing loss, the more a person tends to rely on vision for understanding of speech. Everyone, however, needs to speechread part of the time. In a noisy environment or when listening to poor speech, the normal hearing person uses speechreading, although she or he may not be aware of doing so.

People with mild or moderate hearing losses, who can understand speech with hearing aids, usually depend more on hearing than vision. Still, there are many situations in which their hearing aids do not clearly reproduce speech. Hearing aids are of limited value in a group situation, in noise, or in a room with poor acoustics. Any situation requiring differentiation of speech from any kind of competing signal presents problems to the hearing aid wearer. In addition, many hearing aids do not clearly reproduce sounds like /s/, /f/, /th/, /p/, and /t/. Some people have hearing losses that distort these sounds so badly no hearing aid can remedy the situation. Interestingly, however, these sounds are relatively easy to speechread.

Many hearing-impaired people with mild or moderate losses have difficulty understanding speech no matter how loud it is. Sometimes, the best hearing aid can clarify only vowels but not high frequency consonants. When any of these problems exist, the individual communicates best with a combination of speechreading and aided hearing.

The person with a severe to profound loss may not be able to get enough help from a hearing aid to understand speech well, especially if there is a severe discrimination problem. This individual must depend primarily on sign language, speechreading, or both. Still, anything heard through a hearing aid can help communication even if hearing is not the primary communication channel.

The ability to hear some sound helps speechreading for most people. Even with a profound loss these people, with properly fitted hearing aids, can hear

1. Pauses in a sentence

The individual becomes aware of when someone is talking and where the speaker pauses in a sentence. As mentioned earlier, pauses are very important to meaning. Here is another example.

    a. Goodbye God, we're going home.

    b. Good, by God, we're going home.

2. The difference between long and short words

3. The stressed word in a sentence

The stressed word is usually the most important word. In addition, changing the stress often changes the meaning. For example, **con**tent means what something is about; con**tent** means satisfied. Notice the only difference between the two words is the stress.

4. The difference between asking a question or making a statement

5. Some vowel sounds

All of these features of speech are very difficult if not impossible to speechread. When the audible aspects of speech are put together with what can be seen and understood from context, the redundancy of communication is increased.

A fair amount of research has been done on the effects of hearing on speechreading. Most studies indicate that speech understanding improves when speechreading is combined with listening. Some people are concerned that use of speechreading during early years places too much emphasis on vision to the neglect of hearing. These people favor the use of residual hearing alone during early training of young children. They recognize, however, the value of speechreading once the child has learned to use hearing. With adults and older children, research evidence strongly favors using hearing together with speechreading and/or sign language. For further discussion of these issues, see Berger (1978), O'Neill and Oyer (1981), and Sanders (1982).

What Makes a Good Speechreader?

Although most people can learn to improve speechreading skills, some people seem to have a natural aptitude for it. For a long time, researchers and teachers have tried to understand how good speechreaders differ from poor speechreaders. Although there is still some speculation, most authorities agree that the most important factor in successful speechreading is **synthetic ability**. Synthetic ability means that the person is able to take the limited information seen on the face, fill in the gaps using other information present in the situation, and correctly identify a spoken message. The speechreader sees part of a message, puts it together, and makes sense of it.

In contrast to the synthetic type of mind is the analytic mode of functioning. The analytic person attempts to identify each sound movement before attaching meaning to the sentence, rather than intuitively grasping an idea as a whole. As Jeffers and Barley (1971) said, "The willingness (or ability) to guess and to close is . . . what separates the 'synthetic' from the 'analytic' speechreader."An analytic approach to speechreading does not work because the flow of speech moves too quickly.

Jeffers and Barley (1971) proposed a theoretical model consisting of three factors. The first is visual perceptual proficiency which they defined as the ability to see fine detail and identify speech movements accurately and rapidly. The second is synthetic ability, and the third is flexibility. They defined flexibility as the ability to make quick changes in one's perception of the message if the original decision proves inaccurate. For example, an isolated sentence may look very much like another sentence having a different meaning.

Example A. I have to go.

Example B. I have a cold.

As conversation continues, the speechreader may realize that the first interpretation of what was seen doesn't make sense. If the speechreader is flexible in thinking, he or she can quickly substitute the second possibility which looks the same but makes better sense.

Although the skills of synthetic thinking and flexibility are intellectual or mental skills, they are not related to general intelligence. Analytic thinkers are often highly intelligent people. None of the research studies designed to evaluate the relationship between speechreading and general intelligence have found any relationship between the two.

A number of other factors have been looked at as predictors of speechreading skill. They include

Amount of training. Most authorities feel that the more training a person receives, the better a speechreader he or she becomes. Jeffers and Barley (1971) stated that maximum improvement occurs after one to three years of training, depending on the individual, but that the speechreader must continue to practice if the skill is to be maintained.

Even though most people improve with training, the rate of improvement and the level of skill achieved vary considerably. People start at different levels of skill for reasons we don't fully understand, and they don't necessarily make the same amount of improvement as others in the same training program. There are individual differences.

Therefore, a person in a speechreading training program should evaluate only his or her own improvement without comparison to anyone else.

Language comprehension. Language comprehension means (*a*) knowledge of vocabulary, (*b*) knowledge of grammar, and (*c*) knowledge of everyday and idiomatic expressions. Language comprehension is essential to good speechreading because so much of speechreading involves the ability to use context. Since much of what people see is confusing and ambiguous, they have to use the redundancies or rules of language to decide which one of several possibilities fits into a conversation. Therefore, the better they know their language, the easier speechreading becomes.

Research on deaf children shows positive relationships between language proficiency and speechreading skill. Similar relationships, however, have not been found in adults. Apparently, a basic level of language proficiency is needed for good speechreading, but development of language skills above that basic level does not seem to further improve learning of speechreading. See Jeffers and Barley (1971) for further discussion of this issue.

Duration of hearing loss. It is logical to think that people who have been hearing impaired for the longest time are the best speechreaders because their need has existed longer. This bit of logic is based on the assumption that the need to use the visual channel assures skill development. The research literature, however, does not show this relationship. When speechreading skills of hard-of-hearing adults were compared based on how long they had been hearing impaired, no relationship was found between speechreading skill and duration of loss. Those people who had their hearing losses the longest were not necessarily the best speechreaders. Among the deaf children, the older children tended to be the better speechreaders. However, when language skill was controlled so that it was similar among different age groups, the relationship between age and speechreading ability was no longer seen. What was found was that the better speechreaders tended to be the children who developed their hearing losses after they had learned English. There were, however, many exceptions to this generalization.

Degree of hearing loss. One might suspect that the people with the greatest amount of hearing loss need speechreading the most and therefore would develop the best skills. The research does not show this trend. Simmons (1959) found in an adult hard-of-hearing population that degree of loss did not seem to have a significant relationship to speechreading. Other researchers who compared the speechreading skills of deaf and hard-of-hearing children found that hard-of-hearing children tend to be the better speechreaders (Costello, 1964; Craig, 1964; Evans, 1965; Lowell, 1960). This finding probably reflects the better English language skills of the hard-of-hearing children.

Emotional factors. Most authorities believe that the successful speechreader shows the following emotional characteristics:

  a. Motivation. People who really want to speechread and consider it important tend to progress faster.

  b. Self-confidence. The good speechreader tends to have the ability to accept his or her own mistakes and maintain a sense of humor about misinterpreted messages. He or she does not become upset with communication difficulties but has confidence in the ability to learn and make progress. This person does not hesitate to admit misunderstanding and to use repetition, rephrasing, or other communication strategies.

Costello (1964) found that attitudes among deaf children toward speechreading were important in affecting their skill development. The better

speechreaders were those who (*a*) wanted to speechread, (*b*) felt their parents wanted them to use speech and speechreading, and (*c*) felt their deaf friends had positive attitudes toward oral skills.

Visual skills. Speechreading is a visual skill which is based on the ability to recognize speech movements rapidly. Therefore, it is important for the speechreader to be visually alert and visually attentive to the speaker's face for long periods of time. Visual discrimination—the ability to see fine differences on the lips, tongue, or jaw—and visual memory are also important. Visual memory is a basic part of synthetic ability and flexibility because the visual patterns of speech must be remembered if context is to be used properly. If the speechreader needs to change his or her interpretation of what was thought correct, memory of what the utterance looked like is necessary.

Good vision, with or without glasses, is important for easy speechreading. A person does not have to have normal vision to speechread, however. As long as he or she can see the speaker's face clearly, speechreading is possible. The individual with defective vision, however, may have to make adjustments in order to clearly see the speaker. He or she may have to move closer to the speaker or pay special attention to the lighting in the room.

Summary

Speechreading is a skill involving interpretation of the speaker's thoughts and message. It requires the ability to see speech movements rapidly and to fill in what was not clearly seen by using facial expressions, gestures, the situation, and language context. Speechreading is an intuitive skill, related to good understanding of language. Motivation, self confidence, and the willingness to guess are also important. Although speechreading skill can be learned and improved by training, some people have more of an aptitude for it than others. We know that synthetic ability underlies this aptitude, but we do not know what factors are related to synthetic ability. Intelligence, degree and duration of hearing loss, and educational level do not seem to be related to level of speechreading skill.

Speechreading is an important supplement to hearing, although it is not a substitute for it. The greater the hearing loss, the more the individual needs to depend on vision. Many of the sounds which are difficult to hear are relatively easy to see, and sounds which are difficult to see are relatively easy to hear. Therefore, a hearing-impaired person tends to function best using a combination of aided hearing and speechreading.

2. Limitations of Speechreading

Do you believe that it is possible to speechread every sound a speaker utters and in that way substitute vision for hearing? That is not possible. Even the best speechreader cannot understand every word of every speaker. There are many obstacles to the ability to see all sounds on the face. Some people, however, become so good at using other clues that they understand the meaning of what is said most of the time.

It is as important to understand the problems of speechreading as it is to appreciate the ways speechreading can aid communication. First, a realistic expectation of what speechreading can contribute prevents expecting too much. Expectations that cannot be met often lead to disappointment and discouragement and may cause people to stop trying. Second, when people are aware of the problems of speechreading, they can develop ways to overcome these problems. If they can anticipate difficulty in specific situations, they can plan communication strategies to use in these situations. The subject of communication strategies is discussed in detail in chapter 4.

The Problems of Speechreading

The limitations of speechreading relate to (1) the speaker, (2) the environment, (3) the speechreader, and (4) the speech signal itself. Each category will be discussed in turn.

Problems Relating to the Speaker

Why are some people easier to speechread than others? Lip movements and the amount of mouth opening are very important factors. Some people barely move their lips, and at times they also have careless, indistinct speech that is hard to hear. It is possible, however, to produce speech which sounds clear but is still difficult to speechread. Such speakers are not aware of how difficult it is for the speechreader to understand them because normal hearing people have no problems at all with their speech. People with thin lips are generally harder to understand than those with fuller lips because speech movements are usually less distinctive.

A related problem is nonstandard speech movements. It is possible to produce clear sounds in a variety of ways. When people depend on listening to understand, it doesn't matter how the tongue or lips are placed so long as the sound is heard correctly. With speechreading, however, people learn to associate a particular visual pattern with a particular sound, and when that sound is produced differently, it often becomes confused with other sounds. For example, the /th/ sound as in *this* is usually made with the tongue between the teeth. Some people, however, produce a perfectly good /th/ without protruding the tongue. The speechreader who must depend on what is seen on the lips might easily confuse the /th/ with /d/. Similarly, /sh/ as in *she* is usually quite visible because the lips are rounded. Yet an acceptable /sh/ can be made without rounding the lips, but then the sound is easily confused with /s/. An unfamiliar dialect can create problems because of nonstandard lip movements. In addition, there may be nonstandard use of vocabulary and grammar, further limiting context clues.

It is a fact that limited lip movements are a problem. Sometimes in an attempt to be helpful, a speaker might go to the other extreme and use very exaggerated lip movements. That strategy is no more helpful than minimal lip movement because exaggerated movements distort the speech and destroy the natural flow. The speaker who is easiest to speechread talks a little more loudly and a little more slowly than usual without exaggerating, has clear speech movements, and uses much expression and gesture.

Rate of speech is important. The speech organs (lips, tongue, jaw) move faster than the eye when the speaker is using normal rate. This means that under the best of conditions the eye will miss some speech movements. When the speaker talks rapidly, even more of the speech movements are missed. Slowing down gives the eye a chance to catch up. However, it is not helpful for a speaker to slow down so much that the normal rhythm of speech is changed. Most hearing-impaired people can hear at least part of the rhythm of speech and see some aspects of it as well.

For all of these reasons, a familiar speaker is easier to understand than someone unfamiliar. Speechreaders report that relatives and close friends are easier to speechread than strangers. With the familiar person, the speech habits are known. The specific language structure and dialect are also known, as is the personality. Because these factors are known, it becomes easier to predict the specific expressions that person is likely to use and how he or she makes the different sounds of the language. Even if a person's speech is poor, other people understand it better as they become more familiar with its patterns.

Some people think that deaf people cannot speechread each other because speech is nonstandard. Some deaf people think that speechreading is for understanding hearing people and that the only way deaf people can understand each other is by signing. This is not necessarily true. Some deaf people have standard speech. Speechreading those deaf people is no more or less difficult than speechreading hearing people. Even when deaf people have nonstandard speech, the speechreader can learn to identify their patterns as well as use context clues. Hearing people sometimes find it difficult to understand a deaf person's speech the first time. After listening to that

person awhile, however, the speech becomes much easier to understand. It is very similar with speechreading.

A speaker cannot easily change his or her speech habits, but speech rate is an exception. Usually if a speaker talks more slowly, he or she automatically moves the lips more, projects the voice better, talks a little louder, and sometimes uses more gestures and facial expressions.

There are speaker characteristics that are more easily controlled if the person is made aware of them. One of the most obvious is speaker visibility. You cannot speechread someone whose back is toward you or who is talking from another room. This is one of the most common complaints of hearing-impaired people. Some teachers lecture while facing the chalkboard, not realizing this creates a communication barrier for hearing as well as hearing-impaired students. A common complaint in the home is that one family member tries to communicate with another from a different room. This practice makes hearing difficult even for the normal hearing person and obviously makes speechreading impossible.

A related problem is the viewing angle. A speaker is easiest to understand if directly facing the speechreader. When speechreading has to be done from the side, it becomes much more difficult because there is less information available about speech movements or facial expressions.

Some speakers have bad speech habits such as distracting head or body movements. Gestures related to the meaning of what is said provide additional information, but irrelevant gestures are distracting and interfere with speechreading. The speaker who moves the head up and down or from side to side while talking creates problems for the speechreader. Similar problems are created by the person who moves the hands across the face while talking. These and similar behaviors either cover the speech organs (lips, tongue, jaw) or interfere with the speechreader's ability to concentrate. Any gestures that are not part of the meaning of what the speaker is saying are distracting.

Anything in the mouth of a person who is talking interferes with speechreading. This includes chewing gum, food, cigarette, pipe, cigar, or pencil. The speech movements become distorted under these conditions. Usually the speaker is not aware of what is happening and will not become offended if asked tactfully to remove the interfering object.

Another source of difficulty is the speaker who moves around while talking. Some teachers or lecturers talk while walking around the room. Not only does this practice divert attention from the face but sometimes hides it. It is hard to cope with a moving target.

Everyone probably knows at least one person with enough facial hair to cover the lips. A beard or moustache does not necessarily interfere with speechreading. A problem occurs only if the mouth is partially or totally covered. If the speaker is a close friend or relative, he will sometimes be willing to trim the beard or moustache. At other times, the speechreader must rely more on context when visual clues are obscured in that way.

Problems Relating to the Environment

Environmental conditions can either help or hinder speechreading. Three major factors are (1) distance between speaker and speechreader, (2) the lighting on the speaker, and (3) visual distractions interfering with attention to the speaker. Although environmental conditions cannot always be modified to aid speechreading, often change is possible with some advance planning. Therefore, it is important to be aware of how the environment affects speechreading.

Distance from the Speaker. The farther away the speechreader is from the speaker the more difficult understanding becomes. Most people feel that the best distances are those representative of typical daily conversations—five to ten feet. However, if the speechreader has visual prob-

lems, he or she might need to be closer to the speaker. Distance can be a problem in the classroom, at a meeting, in church, or in the theatre. It is usually not a problem in one-to-one communication. In that situation, however, it is not good to be too close to the speaker because it is difficult to get a clear view of the entire face. It is also important for the speechreader to be on the same level as the speaker, particularly if the two are close to each other. If, for example, the speaker is standing and the speechreader is sitting, the speechreader will have to tilt his or her head back to see the speaker. This head position is very tiring and interferes with understanding.

Lighting Problems. The best situation for speechreading is when the lighting is directly over or slightly in front of the speaker. When the speaker has his or her back to the light, the face is shadowed. Speech movements cannot be seen easily, and speechreading becomes difficult. It is also important that the light not shine directly into the eyes of the speechreader. If the lighting creates a glare in the speechreader's eyes, he or she cannot see clearly. Usually the speaker is not aware of whether the lighting is appropriately positioned. The speechreader should be aware of the problems, however, and ask the speaker to move for better lighting, if necessary.

A sudden change in lighting can create problems because the eyes need a few minutes to adjust. During those few minutes speechreading is difficult if not impossible. The situation occurs any time a person leaves a dark area and enters a bright environment, such as leaving a movie or play and going into the bright sunlight. A speaker who is trying to communicate during that period of time may not be aware of the problem and needs to be informed by the speechreader.

Distractions. Any visual distraction interferes with speechreading because all or part of the speechreader's attention is diverted from the speaker. The effects of speaker mannerisms, irrelevant gestures, and facial hair covering part of the face have already been discussed. In addition, some people find that things in the background make speechreading difficult. Pictures or decorations behind the speaker can distract the speechreader. Similar problems can be caused by some event occurring in the background. Even a bright background can be distracting. Erber (1974) found that profoundly deaf children understood their teachers better when the background was black rather than white. The difference was particularly pronounced when lighting was less than optimal. Background distractions seem to be of particular concern with hearing-impaired children in the classroom.

Auditory distractions can affect speechreading. A number of research studies using normal hearing people have shown decreased speechreading ability in the presence of noise. Berger (1978) summarizes these studies. It is possible that hearing-impaired people who can hear loud noise with or without a hearing aid might experience the same problems. This kind of difficulty can occur at a party, on a job, or in a group situation where several people are talking at the same time. These are precisely the kinds of situations requiring speechreading the most.

Group Communication. Group communication (e.g., at a party, a meeting, or the dinner table) probably creates more difficulty for a hearing-impaired person than any other type of communication for a number of reasons. First, the conversation may jump rapidly from person to person. By the time the deaf individual identifies and starts speechreading the new speaker, some of the information has been missed. Second, topics change suddenly and usually the deaf person is not aware of the change. If the deaf person enters the group in the middle of a conversation, it may take a long time to figure out the subject and most of the conversation may be lost. Third, not all the speakers may be completely visible to the

speechreader. Such situations challenge the normal hearing person. It is no wonder that many hearing-impaired people tend to avoid groups unless sign language is used by all.

Speechreading people on television or in the movies presents special problems. Many people who have tried practicing speechreading in this way have found it very frustrating. It is quite different from live conversation. First, there are rapidly changing camera views on television and in the movies. A speaker may be close one minute and then far away, or a full-face view of the speaker may not be shown at all. Second, not all actors have good speech movements or make a special effort to be completely visible to the speechreader. Remember, it is not necessary to have clear speech movements to be heard clearly. Third, the image on both television and movie screens has no depth as in real life; people look flat. It is much more difficult to get body language clues under those conditions. Finally, the lighting on the actors may not be good for speechreading. For these reasons, television programs do not provide good practice for the beginning speechreader. This type of practice is better for the more advanced speechreader who might choose news programs and televised speeches given by people with clear lip movements.

Problems Related to the Speechreader

As discussed in chapter 1, some people have certain characteristics that make them better speechreaders than others. Some of these factors are controllable. Visual acuity is one such characteristic. Although perfect vision is not necessary for good speechreading, it is necessary for the speechreader to see clearly the face of the speaker. Therefore, it is important that any visual defects interfering with speechreading be identified and corrected. It is also important that a person depending on speechreading compensate in any way possible for a visual defect. The person place himself or herself at the proper distance from the speaker regardless of the situation. If a visual problem is correctable by eyeglasses, the speechreader must always use the eyeglasses.

Visual attention is very important. The speechreader must watch the speaker at all times to follow conversation even though continual concentration is tiring. If visual attention is diverted from the speaker even for a few minutes, important parts of the conversation are lost. People differ in their ability and willingness to concentrate in this manner. Although everyone needs periods of rest from speechreading, the amount of needed rest varies from person to person. The inability to constantly focus on the speaker's face is definitely a limitation of speechreading.

Another problem interfering with understanding is the speechreader's lack of familiarity with the language of the speaker or the topic of conversation. The importance of knowing English vocabulary and grammar has already been discussed in chapter 1. In addition to knowing English, it is important to be familiar with the topic of conversation. An individual will have trouble speechreading when the subject being discussed is unfamiliar. For example, if the subject is the condition of the stock market and you know little about the stock market, you will not be familiar with the important vocabulary and concepts. Complete understanding may not occur even if you have normal hearing, but the situation is significantly more difficult if you are depending on speechreading. If a speaker describes an exciting event reported in the newspaper, the speechreader's understanding is limited if he or she has not read the newspaper. The speechreader needs to be well-informed about topics of general interest as well as topics of specific interest to people he or she associates with frequently. Under standing at a movie, play, or meeting is made easier when the plot or agenda is known in advance.

The attitude of the speechreader is very important. A person will speechread best when the following occur:

1. He or she tries to relax and doesn't strain to catch every word.

2. He or she is willing to guess. Some people just can't allow themselves to guess. They have to be sure of every word. While the speechreader is trying to understand every word, the speaker has continued with new conversation and the speechreader is lost. By the time the introduction to a story has been figured out, the speaker has finished the story.

3. He or she maintains a sense of humor. There are times when a speechreader gets confused, makes mistakes, and feels foolish. If he or she can laugh at an error instead of becoming upset, the speechreader not only helps himself or herself but also the speaker who may become embarrassed. As speechreading skills improve, it is hoped mistakes will become less frequent.

4. He or she is willing to admit when something is not understood. There are many ways a speaker can help a speechreader. However, the speechreader must be willing to ask for help and also tell the speaker how to help. The speechreader must be assertive in admitting difficulty rather than passively pretending to understand. The use of helping strategies is discussed at length in chapter 4, but for now it is important to remember that the first thing a hearing-impaired person must do is say "I didn't understand."

Problems Relating to the Nature of Speech

Speechreading is limited by the fact that, at best, speech is only partially visible. First, normal speech is very rapid. Ordinary speech averages about thirteen speech sounds per second. The eye is capable of seeing only eight to ten movements per second. Therefore, the average speechreader will not see all the speech sounds. When a speaker talks faster than normal, speechreading becomes especially difficult.

Some speech sounds are very difficult to see under the best of conditions. Speech sounds are made when movements of the tongue, jaw, and lips modify the stream of air coming out of the mouth. Many of these movements occur inside the mouth and cannot be easily seen. Some movements, such as those for /k/ and /g/, are totally invisible because they are made at the back of the mouth. Research has shown that, under usual viewing conditions, vision provides approximately one-fifth of the information that is available through hearing (Jeffers & Barley, 1971). Woodward and Barber (1960) found that under usual viewing conditions approximately 60% of all speech sounds are either invisible or difficult to see. Therefore, we cannot rely only on what the eye can see because the eye cannot see enough for clear understanding. This subject will be discussed further in chapter 3.

Many words look alike on the lips. Words that look alike to the speechreader are called *homophenes* or homophenous words. Authorities vary in their estimates of the number of homophenous words in English. Vernon and Mindel (1971) estimated that 40% to 60% of the words of English are homophenous. Berger (1972) looked at a sample of 25,000 words used in conversation and found that 33% had one or more homophenes. Homophenous words are responsible for breakdowns in understanding and may sometimes cause embarrassment. Berger (1978) describes a dialogue illustrating this point.

> Two old friends meet for the first time in several months.
>
> Mr. A: By the way, how is your brother?
>
> Mr. B: My brother was buried last week.
>
> Mr. A: Wonderful! You must be very pleased about that.

Mr. A misunderstood the word *buried* for its homophene *married*. The problem of homophenes

is a severe limitation on speechreading. They can be differentiated only by using context, facial expression, or residual hearing. Sometimes, even these methods are not enough and communication strategies have to be used. For example, the numbers *forty* and *fourteen* look alike on the lips and generally fit into the same context. Differences are also difficult to hear. If it is important to know the exact number spoken, the word must be written, spelled, or perhaps spoken digit by digit (e.g., 4-0).

In chapter 3, the issues of visibility and homopheneity will be discussed in detail, and those sound movements which are possible to see will be described.

Summary

There are a number of problems that interfere with speechreading. These fall into the following categories:

1. Problems relating to the speaker

2. Problems relating to the environment

3. Problems relating to the speechreader

4. Problems relating to the nature of speech

Speaker-related problems include limited lip and jaw movements; nonstandard speech; limited gestures, facial expressions, and body language; fast rate of speech; poor visibility of the speaker; and distracting head or body movements. Environmental problems include improper distance from the speaker, poor lighting, and visual or auditory distractions. Problems related to the speechreader are visual defects, visual inattention, lack of familiarity with the language of the speaker or the topic of conversation, and the attitudes and motivation of the speechreader. Problems caused by the nature of speech itself are (1) the many sounds of speech that are invisible or partly visible, (2) the rapid rate of normal speech and the inability of the eye to function as quickly as the speech organs, and (3) the many words that look alike on the lips and must be differentiated using context.

With all the problems involved in speechreading, it may seem an impossible task. The situation, however, is not as bad as it seems. Some of the problems can be minimized by situational modification or use of communication strategies. Visual limitations can be compensated for by the use of context clues and residual hearing when possible. Because of its limitations, speechreading cannot be considered a substitute for hearing but is a valuable supplement to it.

3. Visibility and Homopheneity

Spoken language consists of a series of sounds that vary in visibility. Although the normal ear can hear more than thirty separate sounds, a much smaller number of those sounds are visually different. Some of the differences that can be heard are based on whether a sound is made with the vocal cords moving (e.g., /b/) or made just with breath (e.g., /p/). Other differences are based on the presence or absence of nasal quality (e.g., /m/ versus /b/). These differences are very important to meaning, but they cannot be seen. The sounds /b/, /p/, and /m/ all look the same on the lips. As discussed in the last chapter, this is one of the major reasons speechreading is difficult. Many sounds, however, are completely or partially visible. It is important for the speechreader to be able to recognize these sounds. There are also sounds which do look different from each other, and the speechreader needs to be able to differentiate between those sounds. The more sounds a speechreader can recognize on the face, the less he or she needs to guess. The visibility of the different sounds of English as well as which sounds look different from each other will be discussed in this chapter.

Sounds of Speech

Vowels

The sounds of speech are divided into vowels and consonants. Vowels are stronger, longer, and generally lower in pitch than consonants and are easier to hear. As a group, however, they are not easier to see. Two major lip and two major tongue positions are involved in making the different vowel sounds. The lip opening may be narrow as in the word *see* or wide as in the word *hot*. The tongue may be raised in the front of the mouth as in the word *she* or in the back of the mouth as in the word *shoe*. Although the lip movements are relatively easy to see, the tongue movements are not.

Most people think there are five or possibly six vowels in the English language—*a, e, i, o, u,* and sometimes *y*. Actually there are many more. In describing vowels, we tend to picture them in a triangle according to the amount of lip opening and whether the tongue is humped in the front, middle, or back of the mouth. Following is a vowel triangle with each vowel placed in a representative word:

Lips	Hump of Tongue		
	Front	**Central**	**Back**
Narrow Opening	see		*suit*
	s*i*t		p*u*t
Wide Opening	s*ay*	s*e*rve	*so*
	s*e*t	*u*p	s*aw*
	s*a*t	st*ar*	

Theoretically all vowels should look different on the lips. However, during rapid speech it is very easy to confuse vowels with each other. Typically, people confuse vowels that are just below or above each other on the vowel triangle. For example, the words *set* and *sat* are easy to mistake for each other. The same is true for *seat* and *sit*. There are only a few vowels that look different from each other most of the time. The vowel in *she* looks different from the vowel in *shoe*; the vowel in *shock* looks different from the vowels in both *she* and *shoe*. Notice that these three vowels are at the extremes of the vowel triangle. The only vowel sounds that look different from each other most of the time are those at the corners of the vowel triangle. Other differences are small and undependable. Therefore, most speechreaders depend on hearing vowels or understanding them from context.

The exact way vowels are made varies from person to person depending on personal habits and where the person comes from. People from different parts of the United States speak differently, as do people from other English-speaking countries. These differences in dialect affect mostly vowels. Therefore, speechreading vowel sounds becomes more difficult when the speaker is using an unfamiliar dialect of English.

Consonants

Consonants are the shorter, weaker, higher-pitched sounds of speech. They are harder to hear than vowels but more important for understanding meaning. Consonants may be grouped in several different ways.

Voicing. Acoustically, consonants may be differentiated based on whether the vocal cords are moving or whether the sound is made from exhaled breath only. For example, the /v/ sound is voiced while the /f/ sound is its voiceless counterpart. Say both sounds and try to feel the difference. The sensation in your throat when you say /v/ is the movement of your vocal cords. The only difference between these two sounds is based on voicing which can be heard by normal hearing people and some hearing-impaired people. However, the voicing difference cannot be seen.

Manner or how sounds are made. All consonants involve movements of the lips, tongue, and jaw, but the way these organs move varies from sound to sound. For /p/ and /b/, the lips come together for a short period of time and then part. These sounds are called *plosives* because there is a very small explosion of air. The /f/ and /v/ sounds are made differently. The upper teeth lightly touch the lower lip and allow a steady stream of breath or voice to escape. A friction type sound is produced which is continuous for a short period of time. Therefore, these sounds are called *fricatives* or *continuants*. The /m/ and /n/ have some nasal quality; they are called *nasals*. Sounds like /w/ and /y/ involve lip and/or tongue movement from one position to another, and they are called *glides*. It is not necessary for the speechreader to learn how all the sounds are made, only to recognize visible differences. Some *manner* differences are

visible while others are not. We will talk about which sounds are easy to recognize later in this chapter.

Place. This refers to the place in the mouth where the consonant is made. Some consonants are made in the front of the mouth and involve only the lips (e.g., /p/, /b/, /m/, /w/). The /f/ and /v/ involve the upper teeth and lower lip. There is a large group of sounds made in the middle of the mouth. All of these sounds involve the tongue and the roof of the mouth, called the palate. Included in this group are /t/, /d/, /s/, /z/, /n/, /l/, /r/, /sh/, /ch/, /j/. Finally, some sounds (e.g., /g/, /k/, /h/) are made in the back of the mouth.

The sounds made in the front of the mouth are usually quite visible. Those made in the middle of the mouth may be partially visible depending on the speaker, the viewing conditions (lighting and distance), and the specific word in which the sound occurs. For example, the /t/ is more visible in the word *top* than in the word *too* because the mouth is more open in the first word and the tongue movement is more visible.

Some consonant movements are not the same all the time. They vary depending on their position in a word and on the sound that follows. For example, /p/ as in *pie* is not exactly the same as /p/ as in *cap*. For the word *pie*, the lips come together and then open. For the word *cap*, sometimes the lips do not open. In the word *shoe* the lips are more rounded for the /sh/ than in the word *shut*. Watch yourself in a mirror as you say these words. Try to notice the differences.

Consonant movements vary depending on the speaker. Most people place their tongues between their teeth when making a /th/ sound, so this sound is usually very visible. However, some people make a perfectly acceptable /th/ sound without protruding the tongue. In that situation, it is very easy to confuse the /th/ with other sounds made in the middle of the mouth such as /t/ or /d/.

Other things that determine how visible sounds are include (1) how fast the speaker is talking,

(2) how carefully he or she makes the sounds, and (3) how good the viewing conditions are. Under usual communication conditions the speaker talks at an average to fairly rapid rate and does not attempt to make very precise movements. Therefore, some of the speech movements that can be seen under ideal conditions, such as in speech-reading class, are less visible. A discussion of which consonant movements are visible under usual communication conditions and which are not follows.

1. The easiest and most stable speech movement is the one for /f/ and /v/, in which the lower lip moves upward and touches the upper teeth. This movement is made by almost all speakers and can be seen even when speech is fast. The /f/ occurs more frequently at the beginning of words and the /v/ more frequently at the end of words.

2. Another visible movement is the one for /w/ and /r/ at the beginning and in the middle of words. The lips are rounded in the "kissing position." Visibility of these sounds varies with the speaker, the rate of speech, and the vowel that follows. Lip rounding tends to be less pronounced in words like *ran* or *watch* than in words like *root* or *wood*. Interestingly, the sound movement becomes more pronounced when speech becomes faster.

3. The movements for /p/, /b/, and /m/ are very visible. The lips move to a completely closed position, are pressed closely together, and then open for the following sound. Sometimes, the lips do not open for a /p/, /b/, or /m/ at the end of a sentence. Notice the movements for /m/ at the end of the following sentence: I did not see him. Similarly, the lips may not open if the /b/, /p/, or /m/ occurs in the middle of a word (e.g., *captain*). The lip movements for these sounds tend to be stable. They are not usually affected by individual speech habits, rate of speech, or surrounding vowels.

4. Another visible movement is the one for /TH/ as in *then* and /th/ as in *thank*. The tip of the tongue can be seen between the teeth. For speakers who do not protrude their tongues, the /TH/

and /th/ sounds are not very visible. Neither sound occurs as often at the end of words as at the beginning or in the middle of words.

5. The fifth visible movement is the one for /sh/ as in *she*, /ch/ as in *cheese*, /j/ as in *joke*, and /zh/ as in *measure*. The /zh/ sound occurs most often in the middle of words and occasionally at the end (e.g., *beige*). The other three sounds can occur in all positions of words. The movement for these sounds involves the lips moving forward into a semi-rounded position. Some speakers use less forward movement than others, especially if the speech is fast. Also, there is less forward movement with some vowels than others. For example, the lips are less rounded in the word *cheese* than in the word *chew*.

All of the other consonants, /l/, /n/, /t/, /d/, /s/, /z/, /y/, /k/, /g/, /h/, and combinations such as /ng/, /nt/, and /nd/ are very difficult to see. They are made inside the mouth with the teeth close together. Rarely can these sounds be identified only by what is seen on the lips; context is very important.

Homophenes

Did you notice that in the description of the movements for the different sounds, there was always more than one sound that looked the same? Because sounds look alike, it is not always easy to identify the specific word a speaker is saying. For example, the words *pay*, *bay*, and *may* look exactly the same. They are called *homophenes*. It is helpful to know which words look alike so that if you interpret a speaker's message in one way and later realize you were wrong, you know which other words are possible. Usually you can identify the correct homophene from the sentence in which it is spoken. Sometimes, however, a sentence can be interpreted in two ways; both homophenes make sense. As the conversation continues, you get more information to help decide which possibility is correct.

Here is an example. First, identify as many homophenes of the word *bus* as you can. *But, bud, bun, buzz, putt, pun, pus, mud, muss* are all possibilities. In the following sentence, only one of the above words makes sense:I want a hamburger on a _____. The word has to be *bun*. In the following two sentences, however, the choice is not clear:

She fell *on the bus.*

She fell *in the mud.*

To decide which homophene is correct, you need more information from the continuing conversation. If you make the wrong choice, realize it later, and need to make another choice quickly, it is important to know what other words look like *bus*. Suppose, for example, you interpreted the statement as "She fell in the mud." Then you saw the following sentence: Two of the passengers on the bus helped her get up. It is obvious that the first choice was wrong and the second possibility is the correct one. In order to switch to the second possibility, however, it is necessary to realize that *bus* and *mud* look the same on the lips.

Now try a homophene exercise. The following words are all homophenes: pie, buy, by, my. You decide which word fits into each of the following sentences:

(1) I like apple _____.

(2) I need _____ book.

(3) I go _____ the library on my way to class.

(4) Please _____ some stamps.

The answers are (1) pie, (2) my, (3) by, (4) buy.

Just for fun, see how many homophenes you can find for the following words: dog, feet, name, shoe.

Hearing and Speechreading

There is an interesting relationship between hearing and speechreading. Some speech sounds that are difficult to see are easy to hear. For example, the vowel sounds are very difficult to speechread, but they are the strongest sounds in

English and can often be heard. Since many hearing-impaired people can hear some or all of the vowels, they don't have to worry about speechreading them. Furthermore, if the vowels can be heard, it is much easier to correctly identify consonants that are not completely visible because there is more information about the meaning of the message.

Some hearing-impaired people can distinguish between homophenous words by hearing the difference. Some people can hear the difference between *man* and *ban* or between *rich* and *which*. Listening can make speechreading easier by providing more information.

Even if a deaf person hears only such things as (1) which word is stressed, (2) whether the speaker is asking a question or making a statement, and (3) when speech stops and starts, speechreading is aided. This information about the rhythm of speech provides linguistic clues to what is seen on the lips, allowing the speechreader to understand better.

Many deaf people cannot understand speech through hearing alone, even with hearing aids. But, if a person can hear some speech and can do some speechreading, the message is understood better than if the person uses only one sense. Every little bit helps.

Summary

The sounds of speech are divided into vowels and consonants. Vowels are easier to hear but more difficult to see, especially if the speaker is using an unfamiliar dialect of English. Most speechreaders depend on hearing vowels or understanding them from context.

Consonants are harder to hear than vowels but are more important for understanding meaning. Consonants made in the front of the mouth are generally easy to see. Those made in the middle of the mouth are partially visible if (1) the speaker is talking slowly and precisely,

(2) viewing conditions are good, and (3) the consonant is followed or preceded by a vowel for which the mouth is open. Like vowels, some consonant movements vary, depending on the speaker and on the sounds which surround them in a word.

Under usual communication conditions the following consonants are visible:

1. /f/ and /v/

2. /w/ and /r/

3. /p/, /b/, and /m/

4. /TH/, as in *then* and /th/ as in *thank*

5. /sh/, /ch/, /j/, and /zh/ as in *measure*

All of the other consonant sounds are difficult to see because they are made inside the mouth. Most speechreaders depend at least partly on context to recognize these sounds.

Many consonants look like other consonants; they are called homophenes. As a result, many words look like other words. We identify the correct word based on whether it makes sense in a sentence or a conversation. Homophenes make speechreading difficult.

Hearing and speechreading work together. Some speech sounds which are difficult to see are relatively easy to hear (e.g., vowels). Other sounds which are difficult to hear are visible (e.g., /f/ and /v/). In addition, speechreading becomes easier if the rhythm of speech can be heard. Therefore, it makes sense to use whatever hearing is available together with speechreading for maximum understanding of speech.

4. Communication Strategies

In previous chapters the many problems that exist for the speechreader were discussed—problems caused by the speaker, problems related to the communication environment, problems caused by the hearing loss, and problems related to the nature of the speech signal itself. In some situations the hearing-impaired person can overcome some of these problems by using a hearing aid and speechreading together. At times, however, the use of hearing together with speechreading does not provide enough information for a person to comfortably follow a conversation. Which communication situations are difficult vary with the individual because hearing losses differ so much. Every communicator experiences some difficult listening regardless of whether the hearing loss is mild, moderate, severe, or profound. Indeed, the normal hearing person has communication problems in certain situations, usually those involving noise or other competing messages.

In this chapter some strategies are described that are useful when speechreading and listening together do not allow adequate understanding. These strategies are not only for hearing-impaired people but also for hearing people when the speaker is difficult to understand for any reason. Chapter 5 presents exercises that illustrate how these various strategies can be used in actual situations.

The Need to Be Assertive

In order to use strategies successfully, a person must be assertive. That means the person must

1. be willing to admit to a hearing problem;

2. be willing to explain the problem to other people when appropriate;

3. be able to suggest ways to improve communication.

For many people the tendency is to try to hide the hearing loss or to make it seem less serious than it is. In that way a real or perceived stigma is avoided. The problem with this approach is that conversation is often misunderstood. The speaker who is not aware of the hearing problem may think the listener is not interested, not paying attention, or not too intelligent. The consequences on the job and socially may be worse than any penalty resulting from admitting a hearing loss.

Admitting to another person that you do not hear well solves only part of the communication problem. Most people do not understand the problems connected with hearing impairment; they think that all they have to do is shout. Yet, the majority of individuals are well-meaning and want to be helpful. Therefore, it is the responsibility of the hearing-impaired person to tell the communication partner what has to be done to make communication possible.

Furthermore, quite a number of people with normal hearing feel insecure about communicating with a person who is hearing-impaired, no doubt because of lack of information. Again, the hearing-impaired person has to be the one to provide the necessary information in a mature, open manner. For example, one might respond to a difficult situation by saying, "I'm sorry, I did not understand what you said because of my hearing loss. It would help if you would speak just a little slower."

In the following pages you will read about various strategies and the situations in which they may be useful. With this information and the willingness to ask for help in a straightforward manner, many difficult communication situations can be made tolerable.

Reactions to Communication Situations

Three ways to react to a difficult communication situation are by being (*a*) passive (nonassertive), (*b*) aggressive, or (*c*) assertive. It is important to know and compare these three types of behavior.

Passive Behavior

The person who reacts passively withdraws from communication situations, thus avoiding real or perceived conflict even if avoiding these situations hurts. Hearing-impaired people may avoid enjoyable social activities, parties, or meetings because they fear difficulties with communication. The possibility of dealing with these problems in a positive manner is not considered. When actually caught in a difficult communication situation, the nonassertive person tends to smile, nod the head, and pretend to understand. Everyone has engaged in this type of passive behavior at one time or another.

There are times when passive behavior is appropriate. Most hearing-impaired people, despite the use of hearing aids, speechreading, and communication strategies, miss some things in some situations. One cannot concentrate all the time without becoming extremely tired. Therefore, many hearing-impaired people decide that there are some situations in which trying to understand is not worth the effort. For example, the individual may decide to avoid noisy parties and choose social activities involving one-to-one communication. The manual communicator may decide to spend a significant part of his or her social life with other manual communicators. The point is that the hearing-impaired person must decide which communication situations he or she wishes to avoid and not have a decision forced upon him or her because of an inability to cope. The individual must not be controlled by passive behavior.

Although passive behavior may be acceptable in some situations, most of the time it results in poor communication. Sooner or later the person pretending to understand responds inappropriately and appears foolish. The person engaging in passive behavior often feels frustrated and inadequate. Self-esteem and feelings of worth suffer. Many opportunities may be missed, socially and vocationally. Truly, a passive approach to communication is not the answer.

Aggressive Behavior

The opposite type of behavior is aggressiveness. The aggressive person expresses feelings and needs openly but in such a way that the other person's rights are violated. The aggressive person is hostile to the speaker, behaving in such a way that the speaker is hurt or humiliated. Aggressive people show bad attitudes. They refuse to admit at least partial responsibility for communication breakdown. Instead the total blame is placed on the other person who may be accused of speaking poorly or doing something to interfere with communication. Sometimes aggressive hearing-impaired people try to dominate the conversation because as long as other people have no opportunity to speak, there is no problem understanding. However, no real communication occurs in these situations.

As with passive behavior, there are situations in which aggressiveness is appropriate. If there is an immediate need to warn someone of danger, aggressive behavior makes sense. In typical communication, however, aggressive behavior results in loss of friends, alienation of acquaintances, and lost opportunities; communication problems are not solved. Good communication involves the co-operation of both partners. An alienated person is not likely to meet the needs of the hearing-impaired individual.

Assertive Behavior

Most of the time, assertive behavior is appropriate for good communication. Assertive people respect their communication partners, but they also meet their own needs. They are honest and open in expressing their feelings and opinions. They admit their problems and ask for assistance. They take the initiative in a communication situation when that is appropriate, without violating the rights of others.

Assertive people share rather than dominate the conversation. They freely admit not understanding, but they also indicate specifically what kind of help is necessary. For example, if the speaker's face is shadowed because of improper lighting, the assertive person indicates (1) the need to speechread because of poor hearing and (2) the difficulty created by the poor lighting. Then, the speaker is asked politely to move to a position where the lighting is more advantageous and is shown where. It is not enough to say, "I'm sorry, I don't understand." The speaker needs to know what to do. Follow up the admission of not understanding by a statement such as, "I can understand you better if the light is on your face." Last, but certainly not least, the speaker is thanked for helping. Most people will cooperate when given information courteously.

The assertive person must know what language is appropriate for good communication. It is possible to be aggressive without appearing that way if inappropriate language is used. Consider a common communication problem. The speaker is trying to converse with a hearing-impaired individual but is not facing him or her. The hearing-impaired person might respond, "What is the matter with you? Can't you look at a person when you talk?" On the other hand, the response might be, "I'm having trouble hearing you because I have a hearing problem. You can help me by facing me when you talk. I'd appreciate that." Which approach do you think will help communication most?

In choosing proper language, there are some tips that might be helpful. First, be courteous even if you feel frustrated. People who try to communicate while looking at something else might be thoughtless, but their cooperation is needed. That cooperation is more likely to occur with an expression of courtesy rather than annoyance. An excellent strategy is to ask the other person to help. When you use the words, "You can help. . . ," you are assuming responsibility for the difficulty rather than blaming the other person. You are also making that person feel good.

The assertive person is ready to use communication strategies advantageously. The remainder of this chapter is divided into sections on strategies dealing with (1) problems related to the speaker or the inability of the hearing-impaired person to understand, (2) problems related to the environment, and (3) problems related to the hearing-impaired person's ability to be understood. The final section discusses some discourse strategies that involve both communication partners and general communication tips for most situations.

Strategies may be divided into two categories, *anticipatory* and *repair*. Anticipatory strategies involve predicting possible problems in a situation or environment and figuring out ways to handle them. They may be thought of as presituational modifications. Repair strategies, on the other hand, involve things that can be done when actually in a difficult situation. These may include things the speaker or listener can do to help communication continue or to repair it when it fails. Both types are important.

Problems Related to Speaker and Speechreader

Coping with a Poor Speaker

You have probably encountered people who speak with food, a cigarette, or pipe in the mouth. Normal hearing people often have problems understanding such speakers, but people dependent on speechreading experience much more difficulty. There are other speaker characteristics that may not prove especially difficult for the hearing person but that complicate the task of understanding for the hearing impaired. These characteristics include speech that is fast, pronunciation that is sloppy, voice quality that is unusual in some way, or speech that is too loud or too soft. A person with a high-pitched voice, such as a child or someone with an unusual accent, may be difficult both to hear and speechread. Generally, an unfamiliar speaker presents more communication problems than a person who is known because familiarity with speech patterns makes them easier to manage. Other speaker-related problems include distracting gestures, limited facial expression, or minimal mouth movements. In addition, a beard or moustache that covers the lips often makes speechreading a formidable task.

Anticipatory Strategies. What can be done to deal with problems related to a speaker? First, it is necessary to identify potential problems in advance, to anticipate sources of difficulty. This is not always possible, but anticipatory strategies can be used more often than we realize. Any time you go into a situation in which the speaker or speakers are known, you can predict the speaker characteristics that are likely to create problems. Once you figure out what is difficult about understanding a speaker, you can plan approaches to minimize the difficulty. Keep in mind, however, that it is always necessary to explain the difficulty to the speaker and tactfully inform him or her what is needed for better communication.

Following are suggestions that may be useful in some situations:

1. If the speaker habitually communicates with something in the mouth, ask him or her to remove the object before beginning to talk. In most cases, the speaker is probably not aware the object interferes with speech understanding. Keep in mind that the success of this strategy depends on the language used in making the request. You want to be assertive, not aggressive.

2. If the problem is soft speech, fast speech, poor pronunciation, or unusual voice quality, ask the person to speak a little more slowly. Often when people slow their rate of speech, other beneficial changes occur too. Distracting head movements tend to slow down or even stop. Words are pronounced more clearly. A person may have more facial expressions and clearer mouth movements. Speech may also become louder when it becomes slower. Some people, despite their efforts and good intentions, find it difficult to slow down, but others do so when they realize the importance of reduced rate. It is definitely worth trying.

3. If you know the speaker, especially a friend or relative, ask him to trim his moustache or beard so that his lips become more visible. It is not necessary for him to remove the facial hair completely, only enough to make speechreading possible. Often the person will oblige; if not, nothing has been lost.

4. The more you talk with a person, the more you get accustomed to a particular pattern of speech. Then the person becomes easier to understand even if he or she has some bad speech habits.

5. There are times when it makes sense to avoid a difficult speaker. If the goal of communication is to obtain information and two individuals can provide that information equally well, plan to approach the person who is easier to understand. For example, if you are aware that certain tellers in your bank communicate better than others, approach the better communicators whenever possible.

6. The person who shouts or uses exaggerated mouth movements probably feels these tactics are helpful. Most people do not realize that loud speech tends to distort lip movements. In addition, loud speech can create discomfort for the hearing aid user. Exaggerated mouth movements also tend to distort speech, creating an unnatural speechreading situation. When aware that a speaker has these characteristics, discuss them tactfully with the speaker, preferably in advance of the communication situation.

Repair Strategies. It is not always possible to anticipate problems. Sometimes, speakers are not known, or unexpected difficulties occur during communication. These are the times to use repair strategies, those strategies that are used during the communication situation. Some of the anticipatory strategies can be used for repair purposes. For example, it is possible to ask a speaker to remove a cigarette or pipe, speak more slowly, etc., while engaged in a conversation.

In addition to the anticipatory strategies used during the communication situation, there are a variety of repair strategies that can be helpful when a message needs clarification.

Repetition. Repetition is the strategy that probably is used most often. It is perfectly acceptable, but it should not be over used. A speaker should not be asked to repeat more than once or twice. Continual requests for repetition will frustrate the speaker and impair communication.

Typically, if a word or phrase is not understood, the listener will say, "Please say that sentence (word) again," or "Please repeat." Other approaches are possible, however. If part of a message is understood, it is good to ask for repetition only of that part not understood. Ask the speaker to repeat the last word or the last part of the sentence or whatever you missed. One way to accomplish this is to repeat what was understood and ask the speaker to supply the rest. For example, the speaker might say, "I met John at the store. " You did not understand "store." You might say, "You met John where?" The speaker knows exactly what is needed and responds with "at the store" or perhaps with "I met John in the store, shopping."

It is good to develop a few key phrases that seem pleasant and use them when you need a repetition. For example, "Please forgive me, I may have misunderstood," or "I sometimes miss an important word or two. What did you say?" It is a good idea to avoid saying "What?"or "Huh?" when a repetition is needed.

Clarification or Confirmation. This strategy is useful when you want to be sure you understood correctly. You either confirm what you think the other person said or ask for clarification. For example, you enter a bus and ask the driver, "Does this bus go to the airport?" The driver answers, "No, it goes downtown." Since you are not sure you understood the last word, you say, "I think you said the bus goes downtown," or "Did you say the bus goes downtown?" If you misunderstood, the speaker will know exactly what you misunderstood and will be able to give you the correct information. If you understood correctly, the other person will confirm your correct understanding. In the above example, the bus driver might respond, "Yes, the bus goes downtown."

Rephrasing. To use this strategy you tell the speaker, "I don't understand what you are saying. Please say it in a different way." For example, the clerk in a clothing store tells you, "I think you would look good in red." You respond, "I'm not sure I understand. Can you say that another way?" The clerk then picks up a red shirt and says, "I think this red shirt would look good on you." This strategy is a good alternative to repetition. It is especially useful when the speaker is using technical or unfamiliar language as in the situation that follows.

A student clinician was explaining a client's hearing loss and used the term *high frequency hearing loss*. The client, who did not understand the terminology, used the rephrasing strategy. She said, "I'm sorry, I didn't understand the last part of the sentence. Could you say it another way?" The clinician substituted the sentence, "You have trouble hearing high pitches." The problem was solved.

Another form of rephrasing is to ask the speaker to expand or "tell me a little more about that." This will provide the listener more information to use to figure out what has been said. For example, a friend has told you, "Our week-long stay in Ocean City was a disaster." After the friend repeats it, you ask her to tell you more about it. She replies, "It was terrible. It rained every day. The place was dirty and the roof leaked. We tried to call the owner, but all we got was an answering machine. The kids both developed colds. It was a disaster." You get the idea.

Sometimes asking a speaker to break a sentence into shorter increments can be helpful. For example, a doctor told a patient, "You have an intestinal virus. You fill this prescription, take it three times a day, drink plenty of fluids, get plenty of rest, and eat bland foods." The patient, not understanding so much information, asked the doctor, "Could you please tell me that again, one thing at a time?" The doctor responded, pausing between sentences, "You have an intestinal virus. Here is a prescription. Have it filled. Take it three times every day. Drink plenty of fluids. Get plenty of rest. Eat bland foods, nothing spicy." The second time, the doctor not only gave the information in increments, but gave some additional information in an effort to clarify the instructions.

Another form of clarification is summarizing. After the speaker conveys a message, you repeat it in a summarized form to be sure the important information is understood. Generally, the summary is prefaced with "I think you said . . . ," or "I think you mean. . . ."

Key Words. Another way to handle a sentence you do not understand is to ask the speaker to tell you the most important word, the key word. If you do not understand the key word as the speaker says it, you can ask for the spelling of the word. If one key word is not enough, ask for the second most important word. A person with good English skills can figure out a whole sentence by knowing one or two key words. Following is an example of how to use this strategy.

Suppose you are looking for a particular person in a building but do not know where he or she works. You ask someone in the hall to help and are told, "He's in the accounting department." Because you do not understand, you say, "I'm sorry,

I didn't understand. Please tell me the most important word and spell it." The other person says, "Accounting department," and spells *accounting*. The message is clear.

Spelling and Code Words. If you have problems understanding a key word, a name, or a number, you can ask the speaker to spell the word. In many instances names of people and places are difficult to speechread. Numbers are often confused with each other and context is of little help. For example, the number 40 looks very much like the number 14 on the lips. One cannot guess these words because precise information is necessary. Spelling frequently clarifies such misconceptions. All you need to do is ask the speaker, "Would you please spell the number or the name?"

If you have trouble understanding a letter, it is possible to ask for a code word to clarify the spelling. You can say, "Was that *a* as in apple?" Prepare a list of code words for each letter in the alphabet to use when necessary. Choose common words you can pronounce clearly. Code words do not have to be used for every letter in the word, only those letters you cannot speechread easily.

Following is an example of how to use the spelling and code word strategies. A person tells you, "I come from Philadelphia." You do not understand the name of the city and respond, "I'm sorry, I did not understand the name of the city. Could you please spell it?" He or she starts spelling *Philadelphia*, but you don't understand the second letter. You then say, "Was the second letter *h* as in *hello*?" Another way to approach the problem is to say, "I didn't understand the second letter. Could you tell me a word that starts with that letter?"

It is possible to spell words by making appropriate finger movements in the air or on the hand if verbal spelling is not understood. If this procedure is necessary, it is the responsibility of the hearing-impaired person to inform the speaker that this kind of help is needed.

Digits. This strategy can be very helpful when you are trying to understand a large number or several numbers spoken together. When you use the digits strategy, you ask the speaker to say each number digit by digit. For example, the speaker tells you, "I live at 144 Elm Street," but you don't understand the number. You can say, "I didn't catch the number. What is the first number?" After you are told the number, you repeat it. Then you ask for the second number and the third. If you do not understand a number as the speaker pronounces it, you can ask for spelling of the number with or without code words. After all digits have been spoken, repeat the entire number to confirm your understanding. Even if you feel that you do not need the number spoken digit by digit, it is a good idea to confirm correct understanding. For example, a clerk at the airport tells you that a ticket costs $125. Since it is important to have precise information, you say, "I think you said $125," or "Do you mean one, two, five?"

Counting. Another useful strategy for numbers is counting. If you cannot understand a number, you ask the speaker to count from zero and stop at the correct number. As this is being done, you count to yourself. Even if you don't understand the person's speech, you arrive at the correct number simply by counting. You can use this strategy to clarify the price of the $125 airline ticket in the following way. You say to the clerk, "Please say the first number." After the first digit is spoken, you reply, "Please count from zero to the correct number and stop." The clerk says, "Zero, one." Then do the same thing with the next two numbers. Finally, confirm the whole number by repeating it to the speaker, "Did you say $125?"

Both the digits and counting strategies are useful for telephone conversation as well as face-to-face communication. Telephone operators know that even for normal hearing people, words, letters, and numbers can be easily misunderstood over the telephone. Therefore, an experienced operator will confirm information spoken by a caller and spell the word immediately after saying it. "Did you say

your name is Jones, J-o-n-e-s?" Code words are used. "Did you say *j* as in Jack, *a* as in apple, etc.?" The digits strategy is used to clarify numbers. "The address is 1-7-0-4 Alabama Avenue." You can use the same strategies to be sure that you understand telephone information correctly and that your speech has been understood.

Writing. Writing is the strategy that makes the most sense in some situations, those requiring exact information. By asking the speaker to write, you will be sure you have correct information, and also you will not have to trust names or numbers to memory. Writing is also appropriate when the other person does not understand your speech. Situations in which writing may be the most appropriate strategy are getting directions; bus, train, or airplane schedules; addresses; telephone numbers; names of people; appointment times; and dates. Writing is also appropriate if all other strategies fail because it is a sure way to keep communication going. Don't give up on other strategies too quickly, however.

In order to use the writing strategy effectively, one must be able to write a clear, easily understood message to indicate what you need. It helps to keep written messages brief, concentrating on key words. For example, if you need the name of a street, you might write, "Street name, please. "

Signing or Fingerspelling. If you use sign language or fingerspelling, it is perfectly acceptable to ask a speaker if he or she knows manual communication and explain that signing will help you. A hearing person will not automatically use sign language even if it is obvious you are deaf. Because some deaf people do not use sign language, the hearing person has no way of knowing whether it is helpful to you. It is your responsibility to reveal that you are deaf and that you need sign language.

Coping with a Known Difficult Situation

Often you can predict that a specific situation will be difficult. Perhaps you know the language will be technical or unfamiliar, perhaps there will not be enough time to use the necessary repair strategies, or perhaps you are afraid that the person communicating with you will be impatient. In addition to these possible problems, you suspect the speaker may have poor speech habits. What are some strategies that can help?

Anticipatory strategies are important here. It is helpful to predict possible vocabulary and dialogue that may occur in the situation. For example, you may be taking your car to the mechanic to have it fixed and feel insecure because you are unfamiliar with the language and the way cars work. This is often a problem for normal hearing people, but the hearing-impaired person has an additional disadvantage because of the speech understanding problem. Although the language may be unfamiliar, it is limited and predictable. In addition, the situation is structured. It is possible to predict fairly accurately the words that will be used, the kinds of questions the mechanic is likely to ask, and the kinds of answers you are likely to receive to your questions.

After you have anticipated the probable vocabulary, dialogue, and questions, you can practice speechreading this language with help from a friend or family member. If you have sufficient hearing, practice listening to the words and sentences. If you are concerned about being understood, practice saying the appropriate language and be sure you can pronounce the words correctly.

You can also take the initiative in directing the conversation. Decide what information you want and what questions you will ask. Try to structure your questions so that the other person can give simple answers using relatively few words. Perhaps yes/no questions or either/or questions will work. For example, you can ask, "Is there a problem with the transmission?" or "Do I need just a muffler or a muffler and a tailpipe?" How you narrow your questions will vary with the situation, but usually you can find some way to do so.

The more specific the question, the easier the understanding.

All the repair strategies should be used as needed. Be sure to have a pencil and paper available for writing technical terms and specific information such as names, times, money, and place locations.

Coping with the Group Situation

There are special communication problems associated with group communication in addition to poor speaker habits and unfamiliar language. In a group, because more than one speaker is involved, the conversation may jump quickly from person to person. By the time the new speaker is identified, some of what has been said is lost. In addition, some of the speakers may not be visible. Another problem relates to the topic of conversation. Topics tend to change rapidly in group communication, leaving the speechreader totally lost. Although a shift of topic may occur in a one-to-one situation, it is far more difficult to get back on track in a group. If a person enters a group in the middle of a discussion, the topic is probably not known. A hearing person is faced with the same problem of catching up with the conversation, but this task is far more difficult when a person depends primarily on speechreading.

Group situations are either social in nature or involve meetings of various kinds. Let us discuss social situations first. One of the most difficult social group situations seems to be the family gathering. The conversation shifts rapidly from person to person, more than one person may speak at the same time, and the subject of conversation may suddenly change. What can be done?

Advanced planning is important. One way to deal with changing topics is to ask one member of the family to be your "cuer," to tell you when and to what the topic has changed. At the beginning of a conversation, tell everyone of this arrangement, and ask for a short delay in the conversation whenever your cuer gives you information.

It is easier to follow changing speakers if each speaker signals in some way before beginning to talk. Perhaps you can ask members of your family to raise a finger before starting to speak. Some hearing-impaired people use a microphone attached to their hearing aids in group situations. The microphone is passed from speaker to speaker as needed. In order to use this device, however, it is necessary to explain in advance how the system works and why you need it.

In order to see the maximum number of people at a social function, advance seating arrangements are needed. To see the most people at a table, it is best to sit at the head or foot of the table. These positions require less body movement to see others. In a living room situation, it is better to sit on a chair than on a sofa. Profile speechreading, which is difficult, is required if people are sitting next to you on the sofa.

These group strategies may be used for any social situation. What is required is prediction of possible difficulties and planning of ways to minimize them. Some of the strategies may be used while actually in a communication situation. For example, if you join a group while a conversation is already in progress, you can ask, "What are we talking about?" or something similar to learn the topic.

Seating arrangements recommended for a social situation will also work well at meetings. The idea is to be able to clearly speechread the maximum number of people. It is best to discuss your plans with the leader before the meeting starts. At that time, explain that you will ask him or her to repeat questions or comments from the audience. If you do not understand what someone is saying, wait until that person is finished, then raise your hand and ask for repetition. In addition, ask the group leader to indicate to you in some way when the topic changes, perhaps by interjecting at appropriate times, "We are now talking about. . . ." Let the leader know before the meeting that you can speechread only one person at a time and that you would appreciate it if all group members

would raise their hands before speaking so that you know who is talking. The group leader sets the procedural guidelines for the meeting and can easily accommodate your needs if informed in advance.

Other useful strategies also require advanced planning. It is always helpful to preview a discussion. Contact the group leader in advance of a meeting to obtain an agenda. If you are attending a course or lecture, obtain notes or a topic outline ahead of time. Some clergy will give a hearing-impaired parishioner an advance copy of the sermon. After obtaining the lecture notes, meeting agenda, or sermon, familiarize yourself with the material. When you know what people are talking about, it is easier to follow a conversation or discussion. You can recognize words and phrases which you might otherwise miss.

Another way to keep up with the discussion is to arrange for a chalkboard or flip chart to be used throughout the meeting. Topics of discussion are written on the board or paper as they come up, as well as important information, e.g., names or numbers. Other visual aids such as models or transparencies may also be helpful.

If you must have a record of the proceedings of a meeting, either arrange for a note taker or ask for a copy of the minutes of the meeting. In a classroom situation, a note taker is essential. It is not possible to simultaneously speechread and take notes. As an alternative to a note taker, you might be able to arrange for the teacher or lecturer to provide copies of each lecture. This may not be feasible, however, because it represents extra work for the teacher.

Use as much written material as possible to help you understand the lectures. Ask the lecturer in advance to recommend books or articles that give information about the subject of the lecture. Obtain the materials and read them before the lecture.

In a classroom situation, ask questions if you don't understand, either during the presentation or later. Ask the teacher if extra tutoring is possible, and if not, consider hiring a tutor. In some places, tutorial services are provided free of charge; in other situations you may have to pay for a tutor.

Consider the use of an interpreter. There are oral interpreters as well as sign language interpreters. An oral interpreter mouths what the speaker is saying, using clear lip movements, gestures, and facial expressions. In that way, the speechreader can understand a speaker who is too far away, is not clearly visible, or has poor speech habits. Sometimes an interpreter will be provided free of charge; at other times the user must pay.

One other area of advanced planning, which may make the difference between understanding and not understanding, is the provision of suitable amplification. Always be sure that some amplification system is available and that the speaker uses it.

Other aspects of coping with the group situation involve environmental factors and will be discussed in a later section of this chapter.

Coping with Television, Movies, Theatre

Speechreading people on television and in the movies is much more difficult than in live situations for a number of reasons.

1. The two dimensional image on the screen results in loss of body language.

2. The speaker's face may not always be visible because camera views and actors may change rapidly.

3. Not all actors are easy to speechread.

4. In the theatre, distance from the actors may make speechreading impossible.

Generally, these communication situations are frustrating. A few strategies can improve the situation, however. Group amplification systems such as induction loops, infrared, or FM devices can be helpful to many hearing-impaired people.

More and more theatres are installing these systems. Hearing-impaired people can form advocacy groups to promote installation of such devices in their communities. In addition, there are amplification devices that can be used with personal televisions. These devices can be used with or without hearing aids, depending on need. Closed captioning is also a possibility, despite the fact that not all television programs are captioned.

For some hearing-impaired people, appropriate seating in a theatre can make the difference between understanding and not understanding. The idea is to sit closed to a loudspeaker. Through trial and error, an individual can find the best seating in a theatre and then arrive or obtain tickets early so that such seating is available.

Finally, previewing a play can be very helpful. Read the reviews or a summary of the plot in advance. You will have a better idea of what is being said and will enjoy the performance more.

Problems Related to the Environment

The use of anticipatory strategies may also include the creation or identification of an optimal communication environment. The following four factors should be considered: (1) spatial relationships, (2) lighting, (3) acoustics, and (4) comfort level.

Spatial Relationships

Your distance from a speaker and the arrangement of objects in a room can interfere with your ability to speechread.

Inability to clearly see the speaker can occur for several reasons. Perhaps the speaker is talking from another room or with his or her back turned to you. In a classroom or at a meeting, a speaker may talk while writing on the chalkboard. Perhaps the distance is too great for clear understanding, or there are physical barriers such as a pole or poor arrangement of furniture. What are some things you can do to help yourself?

You need to think about the situation and predict possible problems such as those mentioned in the previous paragraph. Then you need to figure out ways to manage them. With environmental difficulties, advanced planning works well. Following are some suggestions that may be useful.

First, when a person talks while not facing you or while in another room, that person may not realize that a communication problem exists. It is your responsibility to educate friends, relatives, and others about the speechreading needs of the hearing impaired. It is important to tell people in a polite manner that you must see their faces to understand. People who care will not be offended.

Second, be sure that your vision does not cause problems. If you suspect a visual problem, see your doctor. If you need to wear glasses, always use them when speechreading.

Third, arrive at a meeting, lecture, or class early to get a good seat near the speaker. A good seat is located in the center of one of the front rows. This location will allow you not only to speechread but also to use your hearing most efficiently. If you are unable to get a good seat, perhaps someone will change seats with you if you tactfully explain your need. It is worth asking. If seats are assigned in advance, as for a play, be sure to request appropriate seating as far ahead of time as possible. In order to do that, you must become familiar with the layout of the room, order tickets early, and be willing to explain why you need special seating.

Fourth, discuss your situation with the speaker or teacher in advance. Suggest the best position for the speaker so you can understand most easily. Explain that you must see the face and that speaking while using the chalkboard will impair your ability to understand. Suggest the use of visual aids such as an overhead projector, a flip chart, or appropriate charts and/or models. Explain that if anything needs to be copied from the chalkboard or a chart, you need extra time. You cannot copy information and concentrate on lecture material at the same time. If possible, try to arrange for a note taker in advance. If the speaker cannot arrange for this, provide your own note taker. Still another problem that should be discussed with the speaker or group leader is positioning of furniture. If you feel that rearrangement of furniture can facilitate communication, explain the desired arrangement and ask that it be done.

These simple modifications can make understanding much easier, not only for a hearing-impaired person but also for normal hearing people.

There are things you can do to make the speaker more visible when you are already in a situation. If the speaker is too far away to be seen easily, you can move closer. If the person speaking is in another room, you can either go to the other room or ask the speaker to come where you are. Which alternative is more appropriate depends on the situation and on the relationship between you and that person. If you are communicating with a stranger, it is probably wiser to go to where she or he is located and then do a bit of educating on the need for face-to-face communication. If it is a family member or friend who tries to converse from another room, the matter of who needs to change location should be negotiated.

If you enter a situation and find that the speaker is not facing you, tactfully explain your need for face-to-face communication. This is not difficult to do in one-to-one or small group communication, but it becomes more difficult at a lecture or meeting. It is better to do speaker education in advance, but if necessary you might try it during a discussion. Be sure to be as tactful as possible.

If you enter a group situation and find physical barriers to visibility, e.g., a pole blocking your view, move elsewhere if better seats are available. You should plan for this possibility by coming early, if possible.

Lighting

Proper lighting is very important for speechreading. The light should be on the face of the speaker. If the light source is behind the speaker, it will shadow the face, interfering with the speechreader's ability to see lip movements and facial expression. In addition, there must be sufficient light in the room so that the speaker can be seen clearly, and the light must not be directed into the eyes of the speechreader. How can one improve a situation having poor lighting?

As with other problems, anticipatory strategies work well. At a meeting, lecture, or class, discuss lighting problems with the speaker in advance. Suggest a position where room lighting will best illuminate his or her face. At the same time look at the seating arrangements and find a seat that provides the clearest view of the speaker. Then come early to obtain that seat. If there is some way to manipulate lighting such as using shades or different groups of lights, ask for those modifications before the meeting or lecture starts. If poor lighting cannot be remedied and the room is being used on a continuing basis, try to obtain a room change.

If you find yourself in a situation with poor lighting, tell your communication partner that you are having trouble speechreading. Show exactly how his or her position can be changed so that you can see clearly. Most people will not be offended if asked politely.

If you cannot plan in advance for lighting difficulties at meetings or if the speaker moves around the room while speaking, move quietly to another seat if possible.

Although it is impossible to speechread in the dark, sometimes people don't realize the problem and start a conversation when there is no light. Such individuals need to be reminded to wait until you have adequate light. A situation in which this commonly occurs is at a movie or play. Furthermore, when you leave a dark place for a well-lit one, such as leaving a theatre, your eyes need a few minutes to adjust. Remind your friends

and family that you cannot speechread during that time.

Acoustics

Hearing aids pick up all sounds within their range. A hearing aid will pick up the noise at a party, the cafeteria, or a noisy workplace as well as the speech, making the speech sound muddled. What can be done?

If possible, avoid rooms with poor acoustics such as those having hard walls, tiled floors, no drapes, and no special absorbent materials on walls or ceilings. Such rooms make understanding very difficult even for people with normal hearing. If you go to meetings in such places frequently, ask that the meetings be transferred to a better environment.

Remove the source of noise if possible. Sometimes, you try to communicate while the television, radio, or running water is on. These noises definitely interfere with understanding of speech but are easy to eliminate.

Anticipate sources of noise in a situation, and plan to avoid them. For example, it is best to sit at a corner table in a restaurant to avoid hearing the conversations of other patrons. When making a reservation, explain that you need a quiet place and suggest a secluded corner. Avoid being seated near the kitchen, however.

If you find yourself in a noisy situation and can identify the major noise source, let the speaker know you are having trouble. Suggest that you find a quieter place; to communicate. Sometimes you don't have to say anything. Just move yourself to another place; your communication partner will follow. If you are talking next to a noisy fan, for example, move to another part of the room.

There are assistive devices that can be very helpful in managing noise. Special listening devices such as induction loops or radio frequency hearing aids can be installed in meeting rooms or classrooms. These devices allow the speaker's voice to be made louder than a competing noise. When a group of people are sitting around a table talking, a simple device can often be helpful. Obtain a hand-held microphone and attach it to a portable amplifier with a long cord. Hold the amplifier to the microphone of your hearing aid, and pass the portable microphone to each person who speaks. It not only makes the speech intelligible but also alerts you to who is speaking at a particular moment. Check with your audiologist for more information and plan to use this equipment whenever appropriate.

Occasionally, you will find yourself in a situation where an amplification system is available, but for some reason, the speaker is not using it. It is perfectly acceptable to request use of the system even if the presentation has started. Other people in the audience will thank you for your assertive behavior.

Sometimes noise in a room occurs intermittently rather than continuously. In that situation, it is a good idea to stop conversation when the noise starts and continue talking when the noise stops. For example, if you are near an airport, airplane flyovers can make conversation very difficult. Normal hearing people usually stop talking until the airplane goes by. Remember, communicating in a noisy situation is difficult for everyone, including normal hearing people.

Comfort Level

The comfort level of the environment and the people communicating in it is important for communication. It is difficult to concentrate on receiving a message when the room is too hot, too cold, or too drafty, or when it contains uncomfortable furniture. You should do whatever is possible to resolve these problems.

Expressive Problems

Some hearing-impaired people are concerned about being understood in a communication situation because of unclear speech, incomplete

knowledge of English, or inadequate use of body language and gestures. In addition, some of these people have difficulty writing clear, understandable English. Hearing-impaired people may speak or write messages that can be understood by hearing people who are familiar with deaf speech and language patterns, but strangers may have problems understanding them.

To deal with this problem, the hearing-impaired person must honestly assess each situation in relation to his or her own skills. Then advanced planning can be done. It is useful to identify and practice specific vocabulary that will probably occur in the situation. With the help of a friend, practice pronouncing the words and writing clear messages that convey your ideas. Practice using appropriate gestures to help express your meaning. For example, if you are going to McDonalds, make a list of the foods you might ask for and the phrases you might use to place an order. Practice pronouncing the words and phrases. Write your requests in your best English, and then ask a friend to suggest improvements. Try to predict what the waiter or waitress might ask you, and with the help of a friend practice speechreading those phrases. Think of some appropriate gestures that will help the hearing person understand. On the day you actually go to McDonalds, remember to bring pencil and paper, but try using speech before you write.

All the repair strategies discussed earlier can be used expressively if you are not understood. You can repeat, rephrase, say a key word, spell, use code words, use digits or counting for numbers, or write. You can also keep your sentences short and use words you know you can say clearly. Use whatever is appropriate to keep communication flowing.

If you are entering a situation in which it is important to obtain precise information and you are unsure of your skills, bring along a normal hearing friend to help. Do not underestimate your own skills, however. Use the helper only when necessary.

Discourse Strategies

Discourse strategies that involve both partners in communication are accepted ways to (1) get attention, (2) take turns communicating, (3) give feedback, and (4) terminate a conversation. It is surprising how many normal hearing as well as hearing-impaired people do not use appropriate discourse strategies. Since improper strategies can interfere with communication and send wrong messages to others, it is well to be familiar with generally accepted conventions.

Attention Getting

Socially appropriate ways to get someone's attention include (1) using subtle gestures such as waving the hand or beckoning with a finger, and (2) making eye contact with the other person. No doubt you have seen these strategies used in restaurants. It is important to use appropriate speech to gain another person's attention. Phrases such as "excuse me" or "pardon me" should be used with all communication partners. Other attention-getting devices are (1) gently touching the other person, (2) tapping a surface, or (3) standing up. The first two devices are particularly good with a deaf person who does not respond readily to sound. Turning a light on and off or using a microphone are other ways to alert a hearing-impaired person of the desire to communicate. It is a good idea to inform people with whom you communicate how best to get your attention.

Turn Taking

In good communication, neither partner monopolizes the conversation. Each person needs to be alert to the other person's desire to talk. Therefore, when you are the speaker, watch the other person's facial expressions. When you are the listener, use facial expressions indicating your desire to contribute. Then wait for a natural pause before beginning to speak. In a group situation, raise your hand if you wish to talk, but be sure that the speaker will accept questions during the lecture. Do not raise your hand or otherwise interrupt unless the speaker has indicated such willingness.

Effective Feedback

Good feedback is a critical part of effective communication. Feedback may be verbal or nonverbal. Either mode may be effective for letting the speaker know that the information was received.

Often individuals with hearing loss feel embarrassed when they do not understand. To hide the fact, they will smile and nod, giving a false impression of comprehension. This may lead to further embarrassment or difficulty when it becomes apparent that they did not really comprehend the message. It is the listener's responsibility to provide honest and accurate feedback during a conversation. This may be achieved through the process of *confirmation*, which may take several forms. When you understand information, you may nod your head or say "uh-huh." However, these responses do not necessarily inform the speaker that the information you received is accurate.

A more effective approach would be to confirm by reiterating important points at appropriate times. For example, you might confirm the message, "Okay, we'll talk more when we see each other at Union Station at eight o'clock," by responding, "Okay, Union Station at eight." The speaker then knows what part of the message you have received accurately and what part you may have missed.

Terminating a Conversation

Many people do not know how to end a conversation gracefully. Some acceptable strategies include (1) slowly moving away from the speaker, (2) looking at your watch, (3) politely excusing yourself, (4) standing up, (5) collecting belongings, and (6) putting on your coat. End a conversation with some pleasantry, for example, "I've enjoyed talking to you. Let's get together again soon." If the other person seems reluctant to end the conversation, you need to be assertive but not aggressive. Say something such as, "I'd love to continue talking, but I'm already late for an appointment." Be sure that you are not the person who is prolonging the conversation when the other person wishes to stop. Be aware of his or her termination strategies and stop talking. Do not become a bore.

Some Other Tactics

Be Interested and Interesting. Since current events are often the topic of conversation, be aware of what is happening nationally and locally. Keep up with sports news, popular TV shows, what is happening in your own neighborhood, and your friends' interests. Develop your own interests and hobbies, and share them with your friends. By doing these things, you will be better prepared to understand most conversations you encounter. In addition, other people will want to talk with you and will make an extra effort to help you communicate.

Use Clues from the Situation. Often the situation gives you clues about the topic of the conversation and what vocabulary or phrases might be used. For example, you can easily predict what a police officer might say to you after he or she has pulled you over for speeding. It is also easy to predict what your young child might be saying while pointing to a toy in a store window. A good speechreader uses all the clues in a situation.

Look for ideas rather than individual words. It is impossible to recognize every word in a sentence because too many sounds look alike. In addition, some sounds are not visible, and most conversation is too fast for the eye to catch every word. Therefore, you need to look for key words in a sentence and fill in the rest. If a person insists on recognizing every word, the meaning of the message will surely be lost.

If you interpret a word and later find you are wrong, you need to substitute another word quickly. Suppose you think the speaker is talking about his or her *brother*, but later in the conversation the word *she* is used. The word *brother* doesn't fit, but *mother*, a look-alike word, does. You must quickly substitute *mother* in your understanding of the conversation. This kind of flexibility is very important in speechreading.

Be Observant. Watch everything about the speaker—facial expressions and body language. Most people will raise their eyebrows when asking a question and shake their heads to indicate a negative statement. You can often tell when someone is angry from facial expressions and body position. If a speaker is talking about a particular person, he or she may point to or look at that person. All of this is valuable information.

Be Honest and Assertive. Do not pretend to understand when you are really confused. The speaker usually notices this after a while and may feel that you are not interested in what is being said or may wonder about your intelligence. It is much better to identify your hearing loss to other people and admit when you do not understand. Most people will try to help if you inform them what to do.

Have a Sense of Humor. Even when you make a mistake and feel foolish, retain your sense of humor. Your willingness to laugh at yourself makes everyone feel relaxed and comfortable and allows communication to continue.

Summary

Many strategies that can aid communication in various situations have been described in this chapter. These strategies are summarized on page 35. You may feel comfortable using some; others may not be useful to you. Perhaps you have developed additional ways of coping not discussed in this chapter. Any strategy that works for you is fine. Experiment with the techniques discussed here and any others you can think of. Use what you find helpful. Regardless of which strategies you choose, remember the important things.

- Be honest about your hearing loss.
- Be assertive about asking for help.
- Always think about how you can keep communication flowing.

Communication Strategies*

Anticipatory Strategies:
- Anticipate possible vocabulary, especially new or unfamiliar terms
- Anticipate possible dialogue and its sequence
- Anticipate questions that you will be asked
- Decide what information you want to obtain
- Plan questions you will ask
- Decide how you can narrow your questions
- Anticipate environmental problems
- Plan how you can modify environment
- Consider how you can be assertive

Repair Strategies:
- Repeat
- Rephrase (reword, expand, or summarize)
- Say key words
- Summarize
- Spell key word
- Say each digit individually (for numbers)
- Ask a specific question
- Ask a general question
- Write a brief message (focus on key words)
- Gesture

*Horn, R., Mahshie, J., Wilson, M.P., & Bally, S. (1983, November). *Audiologic habilitation with the hearing impaired adolescent/adult: An integrative approach.* Paper presented at the convention of the American Speech-Language-Hearing Association, Cincinnati, OH.

Listening Strategies

- Ask speakers to speak in a good light and face the listener.
- Ask the speaker to speak clearly and naturally but not to shout or exaggerate articulatory movements.
- Ask the speaker to repeat the message if it is not understood, say it in another way, or use other repair strategies as appropriate.
- Confirm important points or facts by saying them back to the speaker to be sure you received them accurately.
- When entering a group in the middle of a conversation, ask one person to sum up the gist of the conversation.
- If someone is speaking at a distance, move closer.
- If a speaker turns his or her head away, the speaker should be asked to face the listener.
- If conversation is occurring in the presence of noise, try to move yourself and the speaker to a quieter area.
- When in a communication situation requiring exact information such as directions or schedules, it is well to obtain the crucial information in writing.
- Ask the speaker not to speak while eating, smoking, or chewing.
- The person with a unilateral hearing loss should keep his or her good ear facing the speaker whenever possible.
- If possible, avoid rooms with poor acoustics. If meetings are held in such rooms, request that they be transferred to better rooms. Special amplification such as induction loops, radio-frequency hearing aids, or infrared devices are very useful in such situations.
- Request that speakers use microphones.
- Come early to meetings so that you can sit close to the speaker.
- When going to a movie or a play, read the reviews or a summary of the plot in advance.
- In an extremely noisy situation, limit conversation to before the noise starts or after it ends.

5. Practical Exercises in Communicative Strategies

In the previous chapter, various communication strategies were described. This chapter will present practical exercises for situations that we all encounter in daily life and that often create communication problems for hearing-impaired individuals. The exercises are divided into three groups: I. Exploring Communication Behaviors, II. Anticipatory Strategies, and III. Expressive/ Receptive Repair Strategies. By completing these exercises and reading the discussion following each one, you will learn how to use strategies in an appropriate manner.

The first group, beginning on page 38, relates to general communication behavior, particularly how to behave assertively in difficult situations. The development of an assertive way of dealing with communication will allow you to use the strategies described in groups II and III of this chapter. For further information on this subject, see *Effective Communication Strategies: A Guide for the Hearing Impaired** from which the exercises in this group have been extracted.

The second group of exercises, beginning on page 47, will show you how to select and use appropriate strategies before you enter a communicative situation. If you use these approaches, you will have greater influence on the situations themselves, resulting in a greater chance of success.

The third group of exercises begins on page 60. Probably the quickest and most effective way to communicate to others is through speech. Other modes of communication are not as well known (sign language) or time effective (note writing). Hearing and speechreading are used for receiving

information. The amount used of each depends on the degree and type of hearing loss a person has and how effectively the person uses speechreading skills.

Some strategies you might use if you are unable to understand someone include:

- repetition
- clarification/confirmation
- rephrasing
- spelling
- sign/fingerspelling/gesture
- use of key words
- use of digits
- counting
- writing

Either expressively (using the strategy yourself) or receptively (asking the other person to help you by using the strategy) you must be flexible enough to select the strategy which is most appropriate in each situation. For example, the spellings of names vary widely. If someone gave you a name (e.g., of a doctor, insurance agent, etc.), you might immediately ask him or her to spell it rather than repeat it several times (which may not help), or rephrase it (impossible). You should review the last chapter to help you understand the various strategies better.

Two continuums were developed to use as general guidelines for the exercises in the third group: Receptive Communication Breakdown Continuum and Expressive Communication Breakdown Continuum. They should help you to apply these strategies more effectively. The continuums show the different levels of communication that may occur in conversations. Below each level is a list of strategies useful in repairing the breakdown.

---

*Bally, S.M., Wilson, M.P., & Bergan, J. (1984). *Effective communication strategies: A guide for the hearing impaired*. Unpublished manuscript.

If you refer to the Receptive Communication Breakdown Continuum on page 70, you will see that different strategies are used, depending upon the level of breakdown. It is often useful to show how different strategies can be used together to move along the continuum toward complete understanding of what was said. For example,

Given a sentence that is not understood,
"_____,"
a strategy such as "ask to repeat" may be used. Because this strategy is frequently unsuccessful, the sentence still may be completely missed.
"_____."
Another strategy, "ask for key word," might then be used and result in understanding the name.
"Henry _____."
With this information, a "general question" may be posed,
"What about Henry?"
This may result in additional information.
"Henry broke _____."
The rest of the information may be retrieved by asking specific questions.
"What did Henry break?"
"His leg."
"How did Henry break his leg?"
"While skiing."
This strategy has permitted you to obtain the entire sentence. It is then appropriate to confirm the sentence as correctly understood.
"Did you say that Henry broke his leg while skiing?"
"Right."

The communication breakdown has been repaired.

You might use the same approach to help another person speechread you. Refer to the Expressive Communication Breakdown Continuum on page 73. An example of this might go as follows:

You tell a friend about your vacation. Your friend understands nothing.
"_____."
You repeat slowly,
He understands something, repeating it to you.
"_____beach house_____."
You say, nodding to confirm,
"Yes, our beach house in Ocean City."
He understands and repeats,
"Your beach house in Ocean City?"
You say, gesturing toward your wife and yourself,
"Yes, my wife and I are going to our beach house in Ocean City_____."
He understands and confirms,
"Oh, you and Sally are going to your beach house in Ocean City?" You repeat the rest of the sentence,
"Yes, we're going there in July."
Your friend understands.

Study the continuums carefully before you begin the exercises in the third group. You must learn to be flexible! There are many different circumstances that could change the strategies.

I. Exploring Communication Behaviors

Exercise 1. Examining Behaviors

Take a look at your behaviors and how they can affect your relationships and communication with others. Some behaviors seem appropriate for some situations but would not be as good for others. Here are some situations you might experience. Which solution would you choose? Check one for each situation.

A. You are in the beauty parlor or barber shop. You told the hair stylist to cut off two and a half inches of your hair, but he has only cut off a half an inch and has indicated he is finished. You

——————— 1. Pay him, leave, and go back a week later for another haircut.

——————— 2. Explain to him by repeating and finally writing him a note that he misunderstood.

——————— 3. Walk out without paying because he "ripped you off."

B. You live in an apartment with three friends. You wake up during the night because you think you smell gas. You

——————— 1. Roll over and go back to sleep.

——————— 2. Grab your roommates, shake them, and yell, "Get out! Get out!"

——————— 3. Get dressed, knock on a roommate's door, and wait for a reply; finally, you let yourself in and gently waken your roommate to discuss the dangerous situation.

C. Your dentist is drilling on a cavity in your mouth. It is much more painful than you expected. Your mouth is full of tubes and cotton and his fingers. You

——————— 1. Shove him away, remove the things from your mouth, and tell him it hurts too much.

——————— 2. Tap him on the arm and indicate that you need to communicate with him.

——————— 3. Endure the pain and pray that he will finish soon.

D. Your car runs out of gas as you are driving around the campus. You coast into a parking space although it is not in your parking zone. You get a can and walk off campus to get some gas. When you return, you see that a police officer has just given you a ticket. You

——————— 1. Tear up the ticket because it was not your fault.

——————— 2. Write a letter to the campus police, explaining the situation, and asking them to cancel the ticket.

——————— 3. Pay the fine because you know they will not let you register if you don't.

E. You loaned your bicycle to your friend. He returns a few hours later and tells you the bike was stolen while he was in the store. You

———— 1. "Punch out his lights."

———— 2. Move to another room and never speak to him again.

———— 3. Ask him what he plans to do and try to arrange for him to make monthly payments until he pays you the value of the bike.

F. You have just flown back from vacation and have taken a taxi from the airport. As you drive up in front of your house, the driver says something that you don't understand. You assume he was telling you the fare (which you know to be about $8.00) so you

———— 1. Tell him seven times to repeat himself, but you still don't understand.

———— 2. Throw a ten dollar bill at him, get out, and slam the door.

———— 3. Pass him a paper and pencil and indicate with gestures that he should write his message.

Answers and Discussion

The following are suggested solutions for exercise 1:

A. 1. This is not a very effective approach since you have to go back so soon for another haircut and you still have to pay for it.

2. Trying to get your message across so that he can decide what to do about it might be more effective; he may have you remain in the chair so he can cut your hair as short as you truly wanted it.

3. This would probably not be effective because the police might soon be after you. You still don't have what you want, and he's angry at you because you didn't pay him. It's possible that he misunderstood you and his intention was not to "rip you off."

B. 1. This solution could be very dangerous. You might never wake up again.

2. This would probably be the most effective one because it gets some quick action, and the situation could be very dangerous.

3. This solution does not get the action you need in a dangerous situation.

C. 1. If you shove him away you might end up with a drill through your cheek, or do some other damage to your mouth. It's too drastic a way.

2. This gets his attention and gives you the opportunity to communicate. This seems pretty effective.

3. You're still in pain, so you haven't solved your problem.

D. 1. Even though you tear up the ticket, it's not going to help the problem. You'll still be faced with paying the fine which may increase because of the time you'll have let go by. There are also other penalties for not paying a ticket.

2. This seems like the most sensible. If you had a good reason, and you explained to the police, they may reconsider and cancel the ticket.

3. You will continue to be frustrated and angry at the police if you pay it without at least trying

to resolve the problem. You may have to pay the ticket ultimately, but at least you'll feel better and know that you had the opportunity to explain what you think was their mistake.

E. 1. If you do this, he might return the favor. A fight will solve nothing.

2. Taking this approach will not solve your problem. It will not replace your bike and you will have lost a friend.

3. This seems to be the most effective behavior because you're taking some action and trying

to at least give your friend the opportunity to take responsibility.

F. 1. This probably will be frustrating to the taxi driver and may be more frustrating to you.

2. This solves no problem. Perhaps he was telling you not to forget your camera or something else.

3. This will at least find out what it is the taxi driver is trying to tell you without either of you becoming frustrated.

Exercise 2. Identifying Communication Behaviors

Now go back to the chapter, "Speechreading Strategies," and review the descriptions of passive, assertive, and aggressive behaviors. Then read each situation. Think about the behavior of the person described. Write passive, assertive, or aggressive on the line for each situation describing the behavior of the individual.

_____ **A.** Penny entered the office of her boss, the dean. She noticed it was dark and probably it would be hard to speechread. She pushed past the dean's desk (he was sitting at it!) and opened the blinds. Then she sat down and said, "Let's get this meeting over with."

_____ **B.** Wilma replaced the battery in her hearing aid and entered the classroom for the course she signed up for, Feminism in the Deaf Community. She immediately noticed that the room was arranged with desk-chairs in a circle. She was relieved to think that this would facilitate speechreading. However, when the rapid-fire discussions began, she had difficulty identifying which of the 22 participants was speaking. Although she was really interested in the topic, she dropped the course the next week.

_____ **C.** Harry stopped at his instructor's office after the first day of his geometry class. He was feeling really frustrated because he was unable to understand the questions being asked of the instructor by class members in front of him; he couldn't see their lips. The instructor suggested he move to the front row and look back at the "questioners." The next day he was back again. "I still have a problem," he admitted. "I can't identify the speaker quickly enough to speechread. Could we ask the questioners to identify themselves by holding up their hands a little bit longer?" Harry was able to follow class discussions after that.

_____ **D.** Linda was attending meetings in which she was the only deaf person. During the leader's frequent slide presentations, she could not understand what the leader was saying. After looking at the room and thinking about the problem, Linda went to see the leader. She suggested that it would be helpful if he stood near the door during the slide lectures so the light from the hall would shine on him and she could speechread better.

_____ **E.** Gary's computer class was right after lunch. He always felt drowsy and occasionally fell asleep in class. Early in the winter, the teacher said, "I hope the temperature in the classroom is not a problem for anyone. I always turn it up because there is such a draft here in the front of the room." Gary was too embarrassed to raise his hand or complain. Because he missed so much, he got a D in the class.

_____ **F.** Janet's supervisor at work held weekly section meetings to make announcements about work schedules and discuss any problems or special projects that came up. Although her supervisor knew a little sign language, she was frequently in too much of a hurry to stop and translate. Janet was put on probation for failing to report to her shift at the right time twice in one week. She stormed into the executive office and demanded that her supervisor be fired.

_____ **G.** You are late for work but need to stop at the bank before it closes to get some money for the weekend. You give the teller a check. She says something to you that you don't understand. You pass her your pen and a piece of paper and gesture that she write a note. She writes, "ID, please." Soon you're on your way to work with the money in your pocket.

Answers and Discussion

A. Aggressive. Penny's behavior was both rude and demanding.

B. Passive. Wilma didn't try to solve her problem; she gave up on it.

C. Assertive. Harry recognized his problem and worked it out with his instructor.

D. Assertive. Linda analyzed her situation and asked the leader for his help.

E. Passive. If Gary had discussed his problem with his teacher, his grade might have been much improved.

F. Aggressive. Janet knew she had a problem understanding her supervisor but did nothing to attempt to make the situation any better. She did not take the responsibility to find out the content of the important announcements.

G. Assertive. Because you're late you need to communicate as quickly and clearly as possible. You assess the situation and decide that writing is the best communication mode. You are soon on your way.

Exercise 3. Sharing Responsibility

The responsibility for effective communication is on both the sender and the receiver. However, hearing people sometimes do not know about deafness and do not know how they can help you communicate. Therefore, it becomes your responsibility to tell them how to help. Here are some communication situations. Does communication succeed? Why or why not?

Situation A: Kim is in the shoe store trying on some new Adidas. She asks the price. The clerk tells her the price as he ties a running shoe on Kim's foot. Because the clerk is looking down and Kim is deaf, she thinks he does not answer her although he told her the price. Kim then said, "Well, if you won't tell me the price, just take off these damn shoes and let me go somewhere else to shop!" Kim then stomps out of the store. . . .

Discussion: Kim did not succeed. Why?

Because she was rude and demanding. This is called *aggressive* behavior. Other people would rather avoid this kind of behavior and you will rarely achieve your communication goals using this approach.

Situation B: Herb was feeling really drowsy. The temperature in the classroom was so hot he kept falling asleep. Finally, the instructor noticed he was nodding off and said, "Herb, if you can't stay awake, please leave the class." Herb was afraid to complain since everyone else seemed to be wide awake and watching him turn red. Herb slowly crept out of his seat and left the classroom.

Discussion: Herb did not succeed. Why?

Because he gave up too easily. This is called *passive* behavior. If you don't show people how they can help you, a communication situation cannot be improved.

Situation C: Liz was having difficulty understanding the policewoman whom she had stopped to ask directions. She realized her hearing aid battery was dead. She interrupted the policewoman's directions and said, "Excuse me, but I am having difficulty understanding you. I think my hearing aid battery is dead. Would you wait for just a moment while I put in a new one." A few minutes later the policewoman finished giving Liz the directions and she was on her way.

Discussion: Liz succeeded. Why?

Because Liz told the person she was trying to communicate with how she could help. This is an *assertive* approach. She was polite but firm. People usually are happy to help you communicate better if your request is clear and reasonable. (During lunch hours at McDonald's a request to continually rephrase or repeat is not reasonable because it takes up too much time. Writing may be preferable in that situation.)

Conclusion: Although it will not always succeed, the likelihood of succeeding with an assertive approach is greater than with a passive or aggressive approach.

Exercise 4. Selecting Effective Approaches

Read the following situations. Select the appropriate approach for each situation. Check the best solution.

A. You hear a crash in the kitchen. You rush into the kitchen and find your mother on the floor. You call her name but she doesn't move.

_____ 1. You wait awhile to see if she will start to move. Then you call your friend in California to discuss the problem with her. (Passive)

_____ 2. You run outside, grab your neighbor, and pull her into the house to show her what's wrong. Then you shove the telephone into her hand so she'll call the ambulance. (Aggressive)

_____ 3. You run outside, see a neighbor, and try to explain the situation by repeating the problem again and again. She doesn't understand you so you excuse yourself to get a pencil and paper and write a note. (Assertive)

B. The bank has made an error on your checking account. Several checks have been bounced. You go to the bank, which is very crowded, and wait in line to see a teller.

_____ 1. You tell her you'll sue the bank if they don't straighten it out right now! (Aggressive)

_____ 2. You leave the bank when the teller asks you to see a bank officer because you are getting the runaround. (Passive)

_____ 3. You explain the problem and ask to be directed to someone who can spend the time to resolve the problem. (Assertive)

C. You decide to ask your mother to go shopping with you next Tuesday. You walk around the house looking for her. You find your mother and father in the living room. They are having an argument about something very important.

_____ 1. You tell them to stop it; then you ignore your father (who is still yelling) and yell at your mother about the shopping trip next Tuesday. (Aggressive)

_____ 2. You leave the room and wait for a better time to ask since you have plenty of time before next Tuesday. (Passive)

_____ 3. You say, "Excuse me," but since your parents keep yelling, you have to say it three more times. Finally, they stop yelling when your father leaves the room and slams the door. You ask your crying mother about the shopping trip. (Assertive)

Answers and Discussion

In situation A, the aggressive approach is appropriate because it is an *emergency* situation, and you must have immediate results. Knowing your neighbor could have difficulty understanding your speech, you should resort to the quickest means possible to resolve the emergency situation.

In situation B, an assertive approach is appropriate. However, seeing that the bank is crowded, you know that you need to find someone who will take the time to communicate with you.

In situation C, the passive approach is best. It is not polite or a good idea to become involved or interrupt your parents' argument. Being aggressive or assertive will not help, but waiting will.

Although an assertive approach is appropriate and effective in *most* situations, there are times when aggressive or passive approaches may be selected. Think before you act!

Exercise 5. Considering the Consequences

Sometimes it is difficult to decide which approach (passive, assertive, or aggressive) will be the most effective. If you find yourself in this situation, you should *consider the consequences.*

When we act, there is always a consequence or result of our behavior. Some consequences are positive, some negative, and some are relatively neutral. Other people's reactions are important consequences of our behavior and sometimes surprise us. Most of the time, however, we can predict what the consequences of our behaviors will be.

A. Here are some common behaviors for which you can predict the consequences:

Behavior	*Consequence*
1. You reach down to pet a growling dog.	_____
2. You pay all your bills on time.	_____
3. You play the lottery.	_____
4. You get up an hour late on a workday.	_____
5. You get up two minutes late on a workday.	_____

B. You must look at any situation and project the behavior that is *most likely* to occur.

Here are some situations. Write the *most likely* consequence of each.

1. Behavior: You write a check even though you know there is not enough money in the bank.

   Consequence:_____

   _____

2. Behavior: You give your best friend a really nice gift.

   Consequence:_____

   _____

3. Behavior: You park in a "NO PARKING ANYTIME" zone.

   Consequence:_____

   _____

4. Behavior: You buy shoes that are one size too small so they "look better."

   Consequence:_____

   _____

5. Behavior: You forget to water your plant for a month.

   Consequence:_____

   _____

6. Behavior: You buy Pepsi instead of Coke.

   Consequence:_____

   _____

7. Behavior: You buy new socks and underwear when they are on sale.

   Consequence:_____

   _____

8. Behavior: You get a haircut.

   Consequence:_____

   _____

9. Behavior: You do not pay your taxes.

   Consequence:_____

   _____

10. Behavior: You are polite when you ask people to do you a favor.

    Consequence:_____

    _____

Answers and Discussion

A. 1. The dog is likely to bite you.
2. You get a good credit rating.
3. You most likely are not going to win.
4. You will be late for work.
5. Probably very little, if any.

It is possible the growling dog may begin to wag his tail, that a malfunctioning computer can mix up your billing, that getting up two minutes late could cause you to miss a bus and be late for work, or that you might win the lottery and be set for life!

B. 1. Your check will bounce.
2. Your friend will be pleased.
3. You will get a ticket/fine.
4. Your feet will hurt.
5. Your plant will die unless it is a cactus.
6. You will have a Pepsi instead of a Coke.
7. You will save money.
8. You will look and feel better.
9. You will be penalized (fine, possibly jail).
10. They are more likely to do you the favor.

These behaviors had consequences that were easy to predict. It is not always so easy, especially when you ask people to change their communication behaviors.

Exercise 6. Predicting Consequences of Communication Behaviors

Sometimes it is easy to predict the consequences of communication-related behaviors and other times it is not so easy. Here are ten communication behaviors. The first five have obvious consequences. The second five may have several possible consequences. For the first five write the most likely consequence of the behavior. For the second five see if you can write two possible consequences of the same behavior.

1. Behavior: You ask your sister to turn on a lamp so you can speechread better.

   Consequence: _____

   _____

2. Behavior: You ask a friend to repeat the address of another friend.

   Consequence: _____

   _____

3. Behavior: You confirm with the receptionist that your appointment with your dentist is at 3 p.m. next Tuesday.

   Consequence: _____

   _____

4. Behavior: You forget to buy new batteries for your hearing aid.

   Consequence: _____

   _____

5. Behavior: You are watching TV with your cousins who do not have hearing problems and you turn the volume all the way up.

   Consequence: _____

   _____

6. Behavior: You ask someone to give up a seat in the front row so you can see the speaker better.

   Consequence a: _____

   _____

   Consequence b: _____

   _____

7. Behavior: You wake up your roommate because you are not sure if he is having difficulty breathing or is just snoring in a funny way.

   Consequence a: _____

   _____

   Consequence b: _____

   _____

8. Behavior: You do not ask a teacher to repeat a homework assignment because you think you can get the information later from a friend.

   Consequence a: _____

   _____

   Consequence b: _____

   _____

9. Behavior: You pull your car to the side of the road because your passenger is talking to you and you do not know if she is just making conversation or giving directions to your destination.

   Consequence a: _____

   _____

   Consequence b: _____

   _____

10. Behavior: You do not ask your brother to rephrase what he said because he seems impatient.

    Consequence a: _____

    _____

    Consequence b: _____

    _____

Answers and Discussion

Some of these answers may match yours and others may not. Each behavior may have a variety of consequences, some good and some not so good. Here are some possible consequences.

1. She either turns it on or does not turn it on.

2. Your friend repeats the address or does not repeat it.

3. The receptionist nods and says "yes" or shakes her head "no."

4. Your hearing aid stops working and you have trouble hearing.

5. Your cousins get angry, may try to turn the volume down or may leave the room.

6. a. The person says "yes" and gives you the seat.
   b. The person says "no" and refuses to move.

7. a. Your roommate is grateful because you are concerned.
   b. Your roommate is angry because you woke him up.

8. a. You are unable to get the homework assignment from the friend.
   b. You are unable to get the homework assignment from the friend and it affects your grade.

9. a. Your passenger repeats the directions and you continue on your way.
   b. Your passenger says it was not important and will tell you later.

10. a. Your brother continues to be impatient while he repeats what he said.
    b. You do not know what he said and miss some activity with him later.

Exercise 7. Selecting Appropriate Responses

The following are responses to given communication situations where problems have occurred. In the line to the left of each sentence, indicate whether the response is passive, aggressive, or assertive. Consider the consequences of each approach. Then, after each group of three responses, tell which one you would use and why.

Situation A: (To lecturer)

_____ 1. Could you please ask the class if someone in the front row would be willing to change seats with me? I depend on lipreading and my hearing aid, and it would really help.

_____ 2. You have to make someone move! I need a seat in the front row.

_____ 3. Guess I'll sit in the last row and write a letter since there isn't a seat up front.

Which response is the best and why?

_____

_____

Situation B: (To presenter at a meeting)

_____ 1. That overhead projector is blocking my view, but I'll just leave it there because it is too heavy to move.

_____ 2. It would be really helpful to me if you could move that overhead projector. It's interfering with my view of the speaker.

_____ 3. Move than damn projector! It's blocking my view!

Which response would you use and why?

_____

_____

Situation C: (To teacher)

_____ 1. You're no help at all! You're always talking while you face the chalkboard!

_____ 2. I might as well not go to class. You're always facing the chalkboard, so I never understand anything.

_____ 3. You could really help me get more out of our class if you would remember not to continue talking when you face the chalkboard. I depend on lipreading.

Which one would you use and why?

_____

_____

Situation D: (To a person in the audience asking the speaker questions)

_____ 1. Hey! Turn around so we can see your face! I can't read the back of your head!

_____ 2. Would you please repeat the questions for this group? It is difficult for me to locate the speaker and impossible to lipread from behind.

_____ 3. Hmmm, I wonder what the question was. Maybe I can figure it out.

Which is the best approach and why?

_____

_____

Situation E: (At a lecture)

_____ 1. (To friend) The speaker always turns off the lights when she shows slides. I have no idea what the slides are about.

_____ 2. (To speaker) I always cut out when you show slides. I can't "hear you" in the dark!

_____ 3. (To speaker) Could you please leave the podium light on (or window curtain up) when you turn out the lights for slides? I find it impossible to speechread in the dark.

Which answer would you use and why?

_____

_____

Situation F: (In a classroom)

_____ 1. (To teacher) I'm quitting your class! They should never hire a person with a mustache to teach a class with deaf people in it!

_____ 2. (To friend) I quit Park's class. His mustache is in the way, and he is always chewing gum. Besides, he always stands in front of the window when he lectures.

_____ 3. (To teacher) Mr. Park, I'm really having some problems speechreading in your class, and I'm hoping we can resolve some of them. Speechreading is difficult for me because. . . .

Which is the best approach and why?

_____

_____

Answers and Discussion

These are the most appropriate responses for each situation in exercise 7.

Situation A: Response 2 is not appropriate because it is aggressive and demanding. People will be resistant to this approach. Answer 3 achieves nothing. This pas-

sive approach to the situation could easily result in failure in a course. Answer 1 is the most appropriate and probably the most effective response to this situation. The individual goes to the professor in a straightforward manner, explains the problem, and courteously requests a solution.

Situation B: Solution 1 is passive behavior. The individual achieves nothing because he does nothing. Solution 3 is, again, an aggressive approach. Being aggressive and demanding, although it may achieve some immediate results, may result in long-term resistance to helping an individual. In Situation B, 2 is the best approach. Again, it's a straightforward and courteous way of asking for help and achieving a result.

Situation C: Response 1 is an aggressive response. In this example, it is, in fact, insulting. People will be resistant to helping you if you approach them with this attitude. Solution 2, again, indicates passive behavior and will achieve nothing. If you do nothing, you achieve nothing. Solution 3 is really the best of the responses. Being courteous and explaining your needs to an individual who can help has the best chance of achieving the desired result.

Situation D: Solution 1 is too aggressive. Being demanding will seldom get the appropriate result. Solution 3 is a passive solution. The individual is not really dealing with the problem effectively at all. Solution 2 will achieve the best results. Again, it is the courteous approach; it is direct and explains to the individual how he can best help.

Situation E: Solution 1 is an aggressive approach. Complaining to one's friend will not solve a problem when the friend is not even involved. In Solution 2, explaining to the speaker that you cut out of the class does not make her feel that you are interested in the class nor interested in solving the problem. This could be described as a passive approach. Solution 3 would probably be the most effective approach in this situation. The individual talking to the group is courteous and explains clearly what the problem is and how the speaker can best help to resolve it.

Situation F: Solution 1 is an aggressive approach. It's insulting to the teacher and in no way moves toward the resolution of the problem. Solution 2 is not effective in solving the situation either. Quitting a class and complaining about it will not resolve the problems and help the individual succeed. Solution 3 is an assertive approach. It succeeds because it explains to the individual what the problem is, how the problem can be resolved, and approaches the teacher with courtesy and respect.

Conclusion: In most situations, assertive approaches will achieve far more than passive behavior or an aggressive approach.

Exercise 8. Exploring the Components of Successful Assertive Communication

Understanding the Elements of an Assertive Approach

Reread the successful solutions in the exercise on page 39. Can you identify characteristics of successful assertive communication approaches? The following characteristics of an effective assertive approach can increase your chances of success:

1. Courtesy

You are asking the other person to help you. He or she doesn't owe you anything. The nicer you are, the more likely a person is to help you.

2. Explanation

You should explain why help is needed. It helps the other person to understand that he or she is not responsible for the breakdown of communication. It also gives that person the opportunity to assume the appropriate responsibility in the communication situation.

3. Direction

As stated before, a person can't help you if he or she doesn't know how to help you. You need to tell the person what he or she can do to help you communicate more effectively.

Some examples below are more effective than others. In each pair, tell which one is the most effective and why.

A. 1. The man at the information booth at the subway was busy counting change. Beth walked up to the window and said, "Tell me how to get to Bethesda from here." The man said, "Just a minute, I'm busy." Beth waited a long time before he helped her.

    2. The man at the information booth at the subway was busy counting change. Beth walked up to the window and said, "Excuse me, I need some help." When the man looked up, Beth continued, "Could you please tell me how to get to Bethesda from here?" The man said, "If you can please wait just half a minute, I can help you." A few minutes later, he gave Beth the directions she needed.

Which one is more effective and why?

_____

_____

B. 1. Dave told the man at the drugstore he needed some film for his camera. The man turned around to face the film shelves and asked Dave a question that Dave was unable to understand. The man turned around and looked at Dave with a puzzled look. Dave explained, "I didn't understand what you said because I have a hearing problem. I wasn't able to read your lips when you turned away."

    2. Dave told the man at the drugstore he needed some film for his camera. The man turned around to face the film counter and asked Dave a question that Dave was unable to understand. The man turned around and looked at Dave with a puzzled look. Dave said, "Say it again!"

Which one is more effective and why?

_____

_____

C. 1. Darrell stopped to talk with his geometry teacher after getting another D on a test. "I don't understand," said his teacher, "I explained this again and again in class and you still don't do well on the test." Darrell replied, "Because of my hearing problem, I don't understand everything you say in class. You could help me by not talking when you are facing the chalkboard. You see, I really depend on lipreading."

    2. Darrell stopped to talk with his geometry teacher after getting another D on a test. "I don't understand," said his teacher, "I explained this again and again in class and you still don't do well on the test." Darrell replied, "I have a hearing problem and you don't help! It's your fault!" With that, Darrell walked away.

Which one is more effective and why?

_____

_____

Answers and Discussion

Following are the suggested selections and responses for exercise 8:

A. In the first pair of paragraphs, the more successful approach was 2, the one in which *courtesy* was a prime factor. Courtesy is always an important aspect of using an assertive approach.

B. In the second pair of situations, Dave was more successful when he *explained* why he was having difficulty understanding the man in the drugstore. A good, assertive approach gives the individual some explanation as to why communication is not being effective. The better response is 1.

C. Darrell did not take the time to *direct* his geometry teacher as to how he could be helped in the second situation. However, in the first situation, Darrell was probably more successful because he explained to his geometry teacher not only what caused the communication breakdown, but he further directed his teacher as to how to help him to resolve the problem.

Exercise 9. Using an Effective Assertive Approach

Listed below are some situations where you need to be assertive. Using the three basic elements of an assertive approach, write what you would say in each situation.

Situation A: You are shopping for an umbrella. You ask to see a brown one, but the clerk gives you a black one. You say,

_____

_____

Situation B: As you are entering your home, your neighbor yells something at you from the sidewalk. He is not close enough to speechread, and you cannot hear well enough to understand him. You say,

_____

_____

Situation C: Your cousin, Jack, is telling you about his trip to Mexico. He is also chewing gum. You cannot discern the speech from the gum chewing. You say,

_____

_____

Situation D: Someone is at your door. It is your Aunt Tessie. She is sobbing and trying to tell you what happened. She continues to cry, and you can't understand what she is saying. What do you do?

_____

_____

Answers and Discussion

The following are suggested responses for exercise 9. Good answers in this exercise can vary extensively. Check your answers for the appropriate elements of an assertive approach.

Situation A: "I'm sorry, but you misunderstood. I wanted to see the brown umbrella (pointing to the display model)."

Situation B: "One moment, please. Let me come closer so I can speechread you.

Situation C: "Jack, your gum is interfering with my ability to lipread. You could really help me if you'd not chew while you talk."

Situation D: "Aunt Tessie, please sit down for a moment and try to relax before you talk. I'm just not understanding you."

II. Anticipatory Strategies

Exercise 1. Language (I)—Predicting Dialogue

If you plan ahead, you can achieve more successful communication. There is a specific vocabulary and, in fact, predetermined dialogue that can be associated with many situations. In the following situations you will probably find it easy to predict much of the conversation.

You are going to the dentist. You have not gone for three years. You know you have some serious problems. You want to communicate effectively because no one at the dentist's office signs. You project yourself into the situation. What will the receptionist say? Write what you think she will say on the next five lines.

(a) _____

(b) _____

(c) _____

(d) _____

(e) _____

You are shown into the dentist's office. What will the dentist say?

(a) _____

(b) _____

(c) _____

(d) _____

(e) _____

(f) _____

Answers and Discussion

Compare your answers for exercise 1 to these. Are they similar? Are you "in the ball park"?

Receptionist:

(a) Good morning (or afternoon).
(b) May I help you?
(c) Do you have an appointment?

(d) Which doctor are you here to see?
(e) Please have a seat.

Dentist:

(a) Hi (name). How are you feeling? (Dentists often ask this to see if you are nervous or upset so they can make you feel more comfortable.)

(b) When was your last checkup?

(c) Have you been brushing regularly?

(d) Have you been flossing?

(e) Uh huh. Uh hmmm.

(f) Where does it hurt?

Remember this is no guarantee. But the odds are in your favor. The more you can anticipate, the better your chances.

For practice, try some other situations. For example, write anticipated communications for visits to the podiatrist, optician, or other relevant specialists.

Exercise 2. Language (II)—Predicting Vocabulary

Ask a friend to help you with this exercise. Ask the friend to think of a category such as names of friends, fruits, animals, things in a particular room or place, cars, numbers, etc., and make a list of twelve words that fit in that category. Without telling you the category, your friend should start reading the words on the list to you, one at a time, in a very soft whisper or with no voice. You should respond by repeating the word if you think you understand it or by shaking your head no if you don't. Your friend should confirm by nodding if you are correct or by shaking his or her head no if you are wrong. Either way, the friend should move on to the next word.

If you are able to identify the category before the end of the list, your friend should complete the list and then go back to the beginning and review any words you may have missed. If you have not guessed the category by the end of the list, your friend should go through the list a second time. If you are still unsuccessful, your friend should tell you the category and then go through the list one more time.

Exercise 3. Language (III)—Coping with Unfamiliar Vocabulary

Ask a friend to help you with this exercise. Get a map of any state. Have your friend highlight a route that travels from one town or city through eight other communities before reaching another town or city. Then have your friend tell you the names of the towns in a very soft whisper or without using voice. Note how many you get correct. Then look at the map for two minutes to study the route. Ask your friend to repeat the exercise. Note how much your score improves. Becoming familiar with unfamiliar terms can help you prepare for speechreading. Reading a play before going to a performance or reading about a technical topic before going to a lecture are additional examples of using this strategy.

Exercise 4. Language (IV)—Using Constellations

Sometimes situations cannot be as easily anticipated as the dentist. For example, taking your car to a service station for a tune up or repairs. There are many more possibilities as to where a conversation may lead. In such situations, try associating vocabulary with the place or situation. You can do this by making a **constellation**. Diagram a constellation like this.

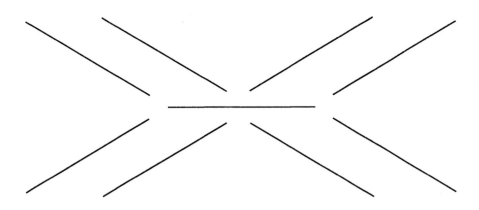

Put the place or situation, such as a service station, in the center.

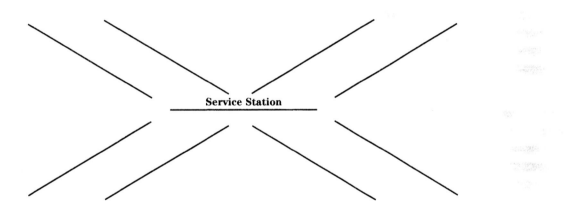

Then fill in the radiating lines with related vocabulary or phrases. Sometimes it helps to close your eyes and imagine the place or situation and write the names of the things you "see."

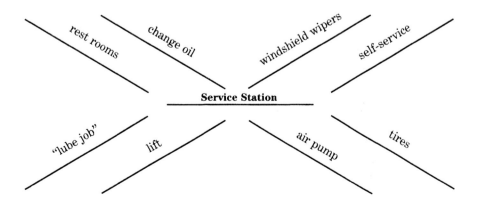

Here is a constellation outline. Try filling in this constellation for a visit to the dentist.

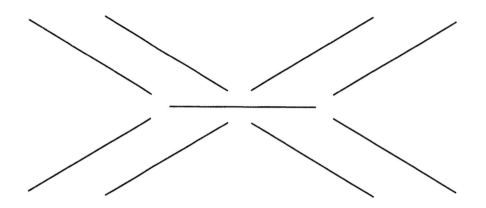

Compare your constellation with this one. Does yours have similar answers?

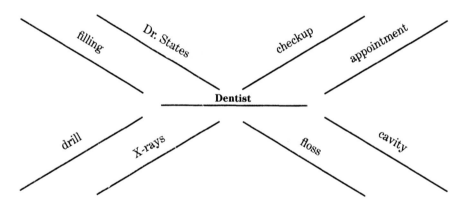

You can do the same thing with people. Here is one I made before I visited my cousin, Harry.

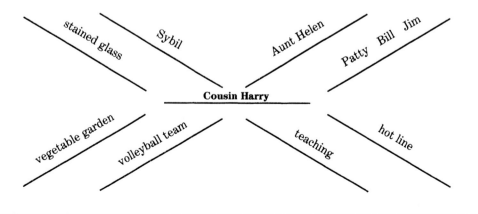

When I think of my cousin Harry, I think of his profession (teaching), pastimes (vegetable gardening, stained glass window making, his volleyball team), service activities (community hot line), friends (Patty and Bill), pets (Sybil), locale and things we have in common (his mother, my aunt Helen and a mutual friend, Jim). I can anticipate when I see him that we will talk about many of these things. I can expect to see the key words which are the words radiating from the center of this constellation.

Make a constellation for your closest friend or a relative you see only occasionally. How will it help you anticipate key words in communicating (speechreading) with that person?

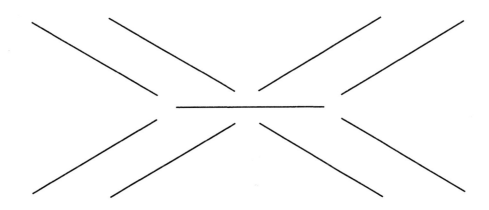

You can also make constellations of things people say in some situations. This will help you to speechread even better. Fill out this constellation with things a shoe salesclerk might say.

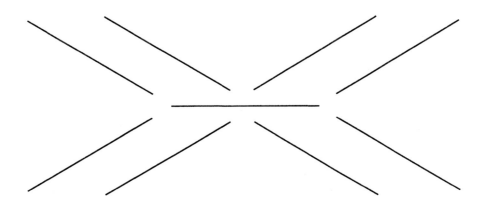

Compare your constellation with this one. Does yours have similar answers?

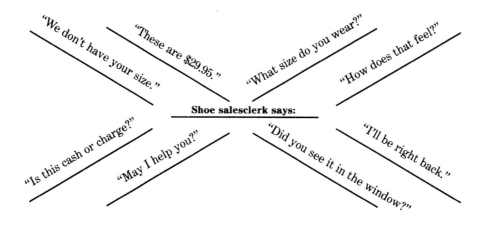

The shoe salesclerk may not use the exact words, but he or she is likely to say similar things. Speechreading them should be easier.

Exercise 5. Language (V)—Controlling the Situation

When you are in control of a situation, you can limit the number of responses that you must lipread. For example, if you are at a bus stop, you may ask another person who also appears to be waiting for a bus when the next bus is expected. There are only three possible types of responses:

a. "I don't know." (or its equivalent)

b. "At 2:00 p.m." or "In 5 minutes" (or other specific time)

c. "In about 10 to 15 minutes" (or other approximation)

The wording may change slightly, but the responses will be limited (a closed set).

In information-seeking situations, the more specific questions you ask, the better chance you will have of understanding the answers.

You are making a reservation for an airline flight for you and your best friend for a Christmas vacation in Florida. What information should you give? What questions will you ask?

1. _____

_____

2. _____

_____

3. _____
_____

4. _____
_____

5. _____
_____

6. _____
_____

7. _____
_____

8. _____
_____

Answers and Discussion

Compare your answers for exercise 3 to these. Did you ask all the questions you needed to?

1. I would like to go to Miami on December 18th or 19th.
2. Which is the earliest flight in the day?
3. Is that the cheapest fare you have?
4. Direct or indirect?
5. What airline?
6. When do I need to be at the airport?
7. When do I arrive in Florida?
8. Can I pay with a personal check?

Some information that the reservation clerk will need includes the following:

- time of departure
- place of departure
- specific destination
- name, address, phone number
- method of payment; if credit card, give type of card, name, number, and expiration date
- travel preferences—coach, first class, smoking/nonsmoking, special diet, boarding problems, etc.

Some questions you might ask include these:

- What is the cost of this flight? Can you get me a cheaper rate?
- What is the carrier (airline), flight number, and time of departure/arrival?
- Will meals or snacks be served?

Each situation will be different. Some things will happen that you didn't expect, but the more you plan the more success you'll have.

Exercise 6. Language (VI)—Asking Specific Questions

When you know you will be in a situation in which you will be asking questions to get specific information, you should consider how you will word your questions. Asking specific questions results in a limited number of possible answers. This makes speechreading easier.

For each pair of questions, indicate which question is better. Explain why.

A.   1. What day is our appointment?

        2. Is our appointment on Thursday or Friday?

Which question is better and why?

_____

_____

B.   1. Are you doing anything tonight?

        2. Are you going to the play tonight?

Which question is better and why?

_____

_____

C.   1. Do you sell electric can openers?

        2. Do you sell kitchen supplies?

Which question is better and why?

_____

_____

D.   1. Is Gallaudet University on Florida Avenue or Massachusetts Avenue?

        2. Where's Gallaudet University?

Which question is better and why?

_____

_____

E.   1. Has anyone been here looking for me?

        2. Has Lydia Frazer been here looking for me?

Which question is better and why?

_____

_____

F.   1. Is the movie at 5:30 or 6:00?

        2. What time is the movie?

Which question is better and why?

_____

_____

G. 1. Do you have Michelob Lite beer?

2. What kind of drinks do you have?

Which question is better and why?

_____

_____

H. 1. What's happening?

2. What are you doing this afternoon?

Which question is better and why?

_____

_____

I. 1. Are there any tickets left?

2. Do you have any tickets for tonight for the balcony?

Which question is better and why?

_____

_____

J. 1. What did Professor Smith talk about in class Friday?

2. Did Professor Smith cover Chapter II in class Friday?

Which question is better and why?

_____

_____

Answers and Discussion

The following choices are the better questions for exercise 4. They are more specific and will limit the number of possible answers. This makes conversation easier to follow even if you depend on lipreading.

A. 2		**E.** 2		**H.** 2	
B. 2		**F.** 1		**I.** 2	
C. 1		**G.** 1		**J.** 2	
D. 1					

Exercise 7. Language (VII)—Practicing Pronunciation

Words are not always said the way they look. This can cause problems with saying words or with speechreading them. The dictionary has a key showing how to pronounce words with which you are unfamiliar. Sometimes they come from foreign languages where letters represent different sounds. Sometimes they evolved for peculiar reasons. Look up the following words and teach yourself how to say them. Even if you are sure you already know how to say them, you might be surprised.

1. quiche	6. island
2. chauffeur	7. massage
3. debt	8. gnu
4. they	9. larynx
5. Wednesday	10. fuchsia

While you were looking in the dictionary, did you look up the meaning of any words you didn't know?

Exercise 8. Environment (I)—Classroom/Meeting Room

Looking analytically at the setting where important communication events will take place can help to prevent some problems from occurring. In the last chapter you read about the possible environmental difficulties relating to lighting, excessive or distracting noise, and the speaker/listener visual relationship. Try applying this knowledge to the next three situations by evaluating the environment in terms of conditions which affect communication.

Look at the diagram and answer the questions following it.

1. Which seat is the best for you? (Circle one) A   B   C   D   E

   Why?_____

   _____

2. Why is seat D *not* a good seat?

_____

_____

3. Why is seat E *not* a good seat?

_____

_____

4. Why is seat C *not* a good seat?

_____

_____

5. Why is seat A *not* a good seat?

_____

_____

6. If all of the best seats with a good view and good lighting and away from noise and distractions are taken, what can you do? (Remember—be assertive!)

Answer:_____

_____

_____

Answers and Discussion

1. If you chose B, you made a good selection. In seat B you have a good view of the speaker, good lighting, and you are away from possible noise sources and other distractions.

2. D is not a good seat. There may be noise from the copier or people in the hall. Visually, the hall may also be distracting.

3. E is not a good seat. You are too far away to speechread effectively. Furthermore, noise from outside the room might interfere with listening.

4. C is not a good seat. You can see the speaker but not the chalkboard. Furthermore, noise from outside the room might interfere with listening.

5. A is not a good seat. You can see the speaker and the chalkboard, but the light from the windows may be shining in your eyes.

6. Discussion:

Seats with a good view of the speaker and chalkboard may be improved if you are assertive enough to ask for the window shades to be adjusted or adjust them yourself.

If the group has not started its meeting, you might ask for a volunteer (or have the teacher ask for a volunteer) to change seats with you.

Remember to arrive at meeting places early so this problem doesn't arise.

Exercise 9. Environment (II)—A Restaurant

You are going to lunch at a local restaurant with some friends. Think about why some seats are better than others for communicating. Study the diagram and answer the questions following it.

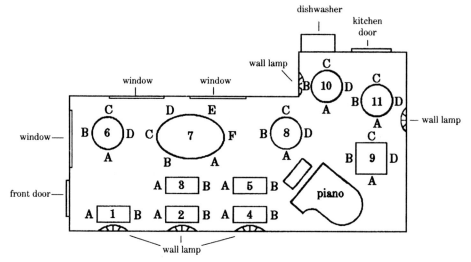

1. Which table would you prefer? Why?

_____

_____

2. Suppose that table is being used. What is your second choice? Why?

_____

_____

3. Suppose the waiter wants to seat you at table 10? Why isn't that a good table?

_____

_____

4. What can you say to the hostess if you see she's going to seat you at a bad table?

_____

_____

5. What is wrong with each of the following tables?

1 _____

4 _____

9 _____

11 _____

6. The host takes you to table 6 for lunch. Where would you sit? (Circle one) A   B   C   D

7. The only table left is 11. Where would you sit at table 11? (Circle one) A   B   C   D

8. You are with a group of six people. The host puts you at table 7. Which is the best seat for you? Why?

_____

_____

Answers and Discussion

1. & 2. Tables 2, 6, and 7 are the best choices (depending on group size). They have better lighting, less noise, and are more removed from traffic than the others.

3. Table 10 has numerous problems. It is close to a major noise source as well as near the busy doorway which could be very distracting. It is not especially well lit.

4. "I have a hearing problem and another table would be much better because. . . ." (Explain reason, i.e., lighting, noise, etc.) Indicating a specific (empty) table would be helpful.

5. Table 1 is close to the front door. The traffic as well as blasts of hot or cold air can be very distracting.

Table 4 is away from the traffic but the sound of the piano may make communication difficult.

At table 9 lighting, music, and traffic may all be problems.

Table 11 suffers from its approximation to the kitchen.

6. B or C. The light illuminates the faces of those people who are with you, making speechreading easier.

7. A or D. The lamp shines on the faces of your companions for speechreading.

8. There are not really any good seats at this table. A and B are the worst because of traffic in the aisle and light from the window glaring in the faces. C, D, E, and F are all reasonable choices, but each has its problems. C and F are close to other tables and far from each other. They are at right angles to other seats resulting in seeing other peoples' profiles which are hard to speechread. A and B as well as D and E have similar problems reading their "partners." It is essential that you be flexible enough to change your angle when you talk with various people in this situation. It would further help if people would signal somehow to indicate when they are to speak so you can adapt your viewpoint.

Exercise 10. Environment (III)—At Home

You are at home or at a friend's home on a rainy Fourth of July. Look at each seat and decide if it would be a good one for communicating or if it would be a problem. Answer the questions that follow.

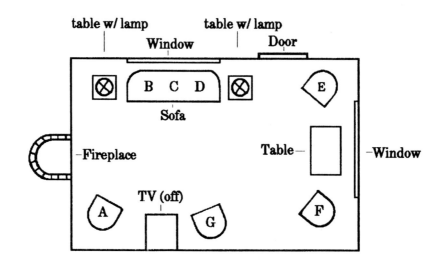

I. Look at each seat. Decide if it is a good seat or a bad seat for communicating. Circle good or bad. After each decision, tell why.

A. good/bad Why? —————————————————————————————————

——

B. good/bad Why? —————————————————————————————————

——

C. good/bad Why? —————————————————————————————————

——

D. good/bad Why? —————————————————————————————————

——

E. good/bad Why? —————————————————————————————————

——

F. good/bad Why? —————————————————————————————————

——

G. good/bad Why? _____

II. If you could move one of the seats to a better place for communicating, which one would you choose? (Circle one):   A   BCD   E   F   G   H

Answers and Discussion

I. This room is not arranged for good communicatio for large groups.

A. Good choice—good general line of vision to sofa; a bit far from G and F; can't see G because of TV.

B. Not bad—can't see E because of lamp on table; also difficult to speechread people sitting next to you.

C. Same as B.

D. Same as B.

E. Bad choice—too far from group; traffic and noise from door.

F. Same as E.

G. Bad choice—can't see A because of TV; can't see F; difficult to see E.

II. Best response: Move A in front of fireplace (not in use of July 4th).

Alternate response: Move E and F forward past doorways.

Other responses:

Move E forward—this may block the doorway and put E's back to F.

Move F forward—this may block the doorway and put F's back to E.

Move BCD forward—sofa is too heavy and move will solve nothing.

Move G forward—can't face A without putting back to F and vice versa.

Optimally, A, E, and F should be moved like this:

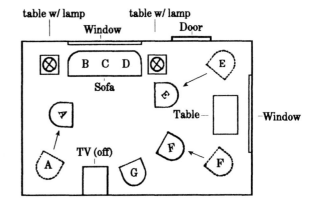

III. Expressive/Receptive Repair Strategies

Exercise 1. Using Receptive Repair Strategies

Study the Receptive Continuum. Then look at the following sentences that someone may have said to you. The blanks indicate a word or words that you did not understand. After each sentence, indicate the point of understanding on the continuum by writing the letter A, B, C, D, or E. Also write which strategy you might choose to obtain the rest of the sentence.

Receptive Communication Breakdown Continuum

Prepared by Barbara Jarboe, Gallaudet University Graduate Student, April, 1984

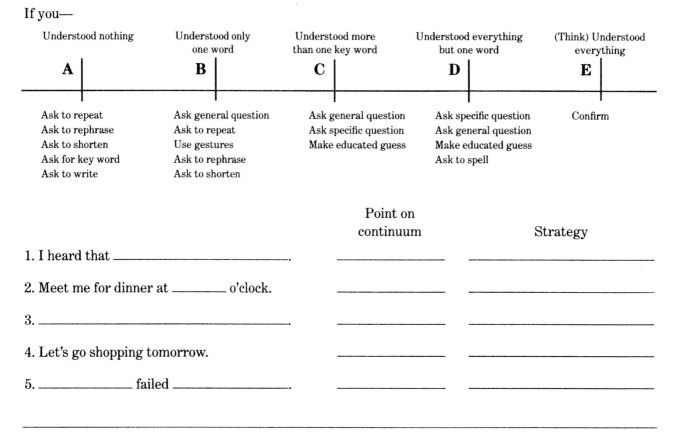

If you—

Understood nothing	Understood only one word	Understood more than one key word	Understood everything but one word	(Think) Understood everything
A	**B**	**C**	**D**	**E**
Ask to repeat	Ask general question	Ask general question	Ask specific question	Confirm
Ask to rephrase	Ask to repeat	Ask specific question	Ask general question	
Ask to shorten	Use gestures	Make educated guess	Make educated guess	
Ask for key word	Ask to rephrase		Ask to spell	
Ask to write	Ask to shorten			

	Point on continuum	Strategy
1. I heard that _____.	_____	_____
2. Meet me for dinner at _____ o'clock.	_____	_____
3. _____.	_____	_____
4. Let's go shopping tomorrow.	_____	_____
5. _____ failed _____.	_____	_____

Answers and Discussion

1. Answer: **C—Ask a general question.**

You should ask a general question to obtain the remaining information. Although other strategies, such as asking the person to repeat what was said, can be used at that level of breakdown, it is better to take advantage of the information you already have by asking a general question such as "What did you hear?"

2. Answer: **D—Ask a specific question.**

As in the first one, other strategies do not make as good use of information already obtained. Even asking a general question ("What did you say about meeting you for dinner?") ignores the fact that you are aware that the missed information is a time. Therefore, a specific question—What time do you want to meet?—is more to the point.

3. Answer: **A—Ask to repeat, ask to rephrase, ask to shorten, ask for key word.**

Because no information was obtained, any of these strategies would be appropriate as a first try. Writing is not included as a correct answer because this strategy should generally be saved for use after failure with one or more of the other strategies.

4. Answer: **E—Repeat for confirmation.**

You may feel you understood the entire sentence. You should repeat the information to the speaker ("You want to go shopping tomorrow?") for affirmation.

5. Answer: **B—Ask a general question.**

Asking a general question works best here because it lets the person know what part of the sentence you understood and what part needs to be repeated or rephrased.

Exercise 2. Rephrasing Words/Phrases

Sometimes people will not understand a word or phrase that you say although you may repeat it several times. It helps to rephrase or change your wording. Can you think of different words which mean the same as the following?

1. infant _____
2. wonderful _____
3. women _____
4. car _____
5. tomorrow _____
6. couch _____
7. bar _____
8. mother's father _____
9. hamburger _____
10. a while _____

11. cat _____
12. kid _____
13. down the street _____
14. friend _____
15. call me _____
16. jot a note _____
17. later _____
18. hurry up _____
19. take it easy _____
20. what's up _____

How can this strategy be used if you don't understand someone else?

Answers and Discussion

1. baby, toddler, newborn
2. terrific, great, swell
3. lady, female
4. auto(mobile), or specific name: Ford, Buick, etc.

5. Tuesday (or whatever it is)
6. sofa, settee, divan
7. saloon, pub
8. grandfather

9. burger, Big Mac, Whopper, etc.
10. short time, few days, few minutes
11. pussy, feline
12. young child, boy, girl, adolescent
13. down the block, road, avenue, etc.
14. pal, buddy
15. phone me, telephone me
16. write a message
17. in a while, shortly, in a short time, in a few minutes
18. come fast, come quick, rush
19. relax, cool it, ease up
20. what's new, what's happening

If you don't understand someone else's speech, you can ask them to rephrase or say it a different way.

Exercise 3. Rephrasing

When people do not understand sentences you say even after you repeat them, you might try rephrasing. Give the same information, but change the wording and phrasing. Here is an example:

"I'll see you at Mark's at 8:00" becomes "You and I will meet at Mark's home tonight. Right?"

Here are some things you might say to people. Think of different ways to express your ideas. Write each one using different words or phrases to convey the same message.

1. "States I would like to visit are Hawaii and California."

   Rephrase:_____

   _____

2. "The answers to the test are b, c, f, b, and d."

   Rephrase:_____

   _____

3. "We'll take the bus to New York. The Greyhound bus leaves at 3:45 on Friday. I'll meet you there. Okay?"

   Rephrase:_____

   _____

4. "When you put fertilizer on your garden this spring, you should use the fertilizer marked 10-20-10."

   Rephrase:_____

   _____

5. "First put in the ice. Then add the gin and a very little vermouth. Next stir gently and then pour into a glass without the ice. You'll have a perfect martini."

   Rephrase:_____

   _____

6. "Dr. Fitspatrick spells his name F-i-t-s-p-a-t-r-i-c-k."

   Rephrase:_____

   _____

7. "When you telephone Aunt Harriet, tell her to bring my records when she comes to visit with you next week."

   Rephrase:_____

   _____

8. "I'm so happy you're coming for Thanksgiving dinner. We'll be eating at 2:00. You can bring the pumpkin pie."

   Rephrase:_____

   _____

9. "In summary, the three principles you need to remember are preplanning, execution, and review. Do you understand?"

   Rephrase:_____

   _____

10. "There is a special movie about Kitty O'Neil on Channel 7 at 8:00 tonight. Be sure that you don't miss it."

    Rephrase:_____

    _____

Answers and Discussion

There are no single correct answers to exercise 3. Any paraphrase which includes the fundamental information is acceptable. Here are some examples of correct answers:

1. "You wish to visit two states, Hawaii and California."

2. "The examination answers are b, c, f, b, and d."

3. "You and I will meet at the Greyhound bus station by 3:45 this Friday. I'm looking forward to going to New York."

4. "10-20-10 is the fertilizer you should put on your garden this spring."

5. "There are five steps to make the perfect martini: (1) Put in the ice, (2) add the gin, (3) add a little bit of vermouth, (4) mix it gently, (5) remove the ice."

6. "The name Fitspatrick is spelled F-i-t-s-p-a-t-r-i-c-k."

7. "When you call Aunt Harriet about her visit next Thursday, please ask her to bring my record albums."

8. Come at 2 p.m. for Thanksgiving dinner. Please bring pumpkin pie."

9. "Preplanning, execution, and review are the three major principles you should remember."

10. "Don't miss the Kitty O'Neil movie on Channel 7 at 8 p.m."

Remember this strategy can be used if you don't understand someone else. Simply request in a polite way that they say it a different way or rephrase it.

Exercise 4. Additional Rephrasing Strategies

Incrementing, expanding, and summarizing are three helpful modifications of the rephrasing strategy. *Incrementing* means asking the speaker to break up or separate the message into shorter sentences or phrases. *Expanding* means asking the speaker to expand upon the message so you receive more information. *Summarizing* means making the message shorter, giving only the essential information.

A. Increment the next five sentences by breaking them into smaller sentences.

1. Take Route 54 about five miles until you see a hospital on your left and turn right at the next intersection on Old Woodmont Road.

   Increment:_____

   _____

2. Mom will bring the honey-glazed baked ham, Lucy will make some macaroni salad, and I'll bring the beverages.

   Increment:_____

   _____

3. Mix 1 cup of sugar, 1 cup of vegetable oil, 3 cups of flour, 2 eggs, well beaten, a teaspoon of vanilla, and chop in 1/4 pound of softened butter.

   Increment:_____

   _____

4. Okay, I'm reviewing this information and your credit card number is 0067-1207-5409-3171, expiring 10-97, and your mailing address is 77 Sunset Strip in St. Louis, Missouri, zip code 63177.

   Increment:_____

   _____

5. We'll be in Phoenix for two days on Thursday and Friday, drive to Albuquerque on Saturday and stay till Tuesday, then drive to Santa Fe Wednesday morning for three days and finish up at Taos for the weekend.

   Increment:_____

   _____

B. Expand on the next five sentences to show how a speaker might help a listener understand better. You may make up additional information if you want.

1. Bob fractured his ulna.

   Expand:_____

   _____

2. How many deductions did you claim on your income taxes?

   Expand:_____

   _____

3. Salt air may cause your padlock to oxidize and seize up.

   Expand:_____

   _____

4. You'll need to complete the registration process next Monday.

   Expand:_____

   _____

5. You need to enrich your soil.

   Expand:_____

   _____

C. Summarize the next five sentences to help a listener understand.

1. Bring the damaged mantel clock to the claims counter with the damaged merchandise claims form we mailed you and ask for Ms. McLagan.

   Summarize:_____

   _____

2. I'm really looking forward to seeing you at the beach as close to noon as possible, when we meet next Thursday in front of the pizza shop at the end of Balitmore Avenue.

   Summarize:_____

   _____

3. I'd like a bacon, lettuce, and tomato sandwich on toasted rye bread with mayonnaise, please.

   Summarize:_____

   _____

4. Let me make sure your order is correct—you want two pairs of the bedroom slippers, as shown on page 42 of the catalogue in green in a size 8 and the "Cherokee Dawn" pullover shown on page 67 in a size medium.

Summarize:_____

_____

5. Please make fourteen copies of the report, put the pages in numerical order, staple them, and put each one in an envelope with each of the board member's names on them.

Summarize:_____

_____

Answers and Discussions

Your answers should be similar to the ones that follow. You may review these as examples.

A. 1. Take Route 54 for about five miles. You will see a hospital on your left. Turn right at the next intersection. You will turn onto Old Woodmont Road.

2. Mom will bring the honey-glazed baked ham. Lucy will make some macaroni salad. I'll bring the beverages.

3. Mix 1 cup of sugar. One cup of vegetable oil. Three cups of flour. Two eggs, well beaten. A teaspoon of vanilla. Then chop in 1/4 cup of softened butter.

4. Okay, let's review your card number and address. Your credit card number is 0067-1207-5409-3171. It expires in October 1997. Your mailing address is 77 Sunset Strip. That's in St. Louis, Missouri. Your zip code is 63177.

5. We'll be in Phoenix for two days on Thursday and Friday. We drive to Albuqerque on Saturday and stay till Tuesday. Then we drive to Santa Fe on Wednesday morning for three days. Then we finish up at Taos for the weekend.

B. 1. Bob fell and hurt his arm. He fractured a bone. It was the ulna bone.

2. Did you finish your income taxes this year? Did you claim any deductions? How many did you take?

3. Be careful of using a padlock at the beach. The salt air is bad for metal. It may cause your padlock to oxidize. If your padlock oxidizes, the parts may stop moving. It may seize up.

4. Next Monday you will need to come to campus. You will need to sign up for your course. First see your advisor for the registration forms. Then go to the Finance Office to pay. Then go to the Registrar's Office to turn in the paperwork.

5. The soil in your garden seems weak. The flowers are not doing well. You can add things to the dirt to make it better. You can mix in manure, some sand, and peat moss. That will enrich the soil.

C. 1. Bring the clock and the claims form to the claims counter and ask for Ms. McLagan.

2. We will meet next Thursday at noon at the pizza shop on Baltimore Avenue.

3. A B-L-T on rye toast with mayonnaise, please.

4. You want two pairs of the green bedroom slippers, size 8, shown on page 42. You want the Cherokee Dawn pullover, size medium, from page 67.

5. Please make fourteen collated, stapled copies of the report and put them in labeled envelopes for each board member.

Exercise 5. Key Words

Determining the key words is important for both speaking (and note writing) and listening/speechreading. Frequently the key words are the nouns, verbs, prepositions, and direct objects in a sentence. These include proper names, dates, times, and other important information. In each question or statement, underline the key words.

1. I've been looking all over for Cindy, but I can't find her. Where did Cindy go this afternoon?

2. I'd like to plan ahead, so tell me when we are going to the movie tonight.

3. When Jim Dyck was traveling this year, he stopped in Huntington Beach, California.

4. I hope you will remember to buy some toothpaste while you are at the shopping mall this afternoon.

5. Who is the lady who won the tennis match for the fourth time in two years?

6. How many miles is it before we get to the town of Wilmington?

7. Our little baby, who is usually so healthy, had a 102° temperature last night.

8. Gary is so very thoughtful. He remembered to bring me some really lovely roses for my birthday celebration.

9. I've been thinking that I'd like to sign up for an economics class in the fall of 1984.

10. This weekend, one of the movies that I really want to rent is "Casablanca."

Answers and Discussion

Each sentence is repeated here. The words that are most important are the key words. They are underlined twice. You should have underlined all of these. There are some other important words in each sentence. They are underlined once. If you underlined these as well, that's fine because they are important.

1. I've been <u>looking</u> all over <u>for Cindy</u>, but I <u>can't find</u> her. <u>Where</u> did <u>Cindy go</u> this <u>afternoon</u>?

2. I'd like to plan ahead, so tell me <u>when</u> we are <u>going</u> to the <u>movie tonight</u>.

3. When <u>Jim Dyck</u> was traveling this year, he <u>stopped</u> in <u>Huntington Beach, California</u>.

4. I hope you will remember to <u>buy</u> some <u>toothpaste</u> while you are at the <u>shopping</u> mall <u>this afternoon</u>.

5. <u>Who</u> is the lady who <u>won</u> the <u>tennis match</u> for the fourth time in two years?

6. <u>How many miles</u> is it before we get <u>to</u> the town of <u>Wilmington</u>?

7. Our little <u>baby</u>, who is usually so healthy, had a <u>102° temperature last night</u>.

8. <u>Gary</u> is to very <u>thoughtful</u>. He remembered to <u>bring</u> me some really lovely <u>roses for</u> my <u>birthday</u> celebration.

9. I've been thinking that <u>I'd like</u> to sign up for an <u>economics class</u> in the <u>fall</u> of <u>1984</u>.

10. This weekend, <u>one</u> of the <u>movies</u> that I <u>really want</u> to <u>rent</u> is "<u>Casablanca</u>."

Exercise 6. Notewriting with Key Words

In the last exercise, you underlined the key words. Key words can be used to write *concise* notes. Here are the key words from the first two sentences in the last exercise:

Where   Cindy   go?

When   we   go   movie   tonight?

These notes using key words are brief but give all the necessary information.

A.   What is wrong with the following notes?

1. need 3, here 2

    Problem: _____

2. 3 o'clock train?

    Problem: _____

3. bring with you?

    Problem: _____

When you write a note, if it is a question, you should always include the question word (who, what, when, etc., except verbs of being—are, is, am).

Example:

When you come?

Why Paul late?

Where money?

B.   Write a note for each of these questions.

1. Who is coming for dinner Wednesday night?

    Note: _____

2. When does your *Time* magazine subscription expire?

    Note: _____

3. When is your appointment with the dentist?

    Note: _____

4. What tools will you bring with you to fix the car?

    Note: _____

5. How are you planning to get to Florida?

    Note: _____

6. Where do you think you will go for your vacation this August?

    Note: _____

7. Why did your professor fail you in his geology course?

    Note: _____

8. Who broke the lamp that was over there by the door?

    Note: _____

9. What was the doctor's diagnosis of your illness?

    Note: _____

10. Where do you keep all of your history notes?

    Note: _____

Answers and Discussion

There are many times when note writing is the most efficient strategy for communication. But, to succeed notes must be clear and concise.

A. 1. This note says that 3 are needed but does not tell 3 of what! It also does not tell who needs 3.

   2. This note asks something about a 3 o'clock train, but it doesn't tell if it wants to know where it is, when it's coming, or anything.

   3. This note is about bringing something with you, but it never says what!

3. When your dentist appointment?
4. What tools bring fix car?
5. How you getting to Florida?
6. Where you go vacation August?
7. Why professor fail you geology?
8. Who broke lamp by door?
9. What doctor's diagnosis?
10. Where keep history notes?

B. 1. Who coming Wednesday dinner?

   2. When *Time* subscription expire?

Exercise 7. Using Confirmation as a Strategy

Key words can be used effectively in the expressive strategies described as "clarification or confirmation." For example, your friend says, "I will call you Friday at 7:00 p.m." The key words are *call, Friday, 7:00 p.m.* These can be used to phrase a response such as "I look forward to your call Friday at 7:00," or "I'll expect your call at 7:00 on Friday."

In the following sentences, first underline the key words. Then using the key words, write a response which confirms the information you perceived.

1. The plane that John is taking to Arizona arrives in Tucson at 6:40 in the morning.

   Response:_____

2. Tell Brian that his Cousin Betty had twins last Thursday.

   Response:_____

   _____

3. I checked the bulletin board this afternoon, and your score for the physics mid-term was 93.

   Response:_____

   _____

4. Next month, in September, Harry and I are planning to go on a trip to Kenya.

   Response:_____

   _____

5. The people who came to tryouts that I have selected for the team are Darrell, Ron, and David.

   Response:_____

   _____

6. No, no! That wasn't one cup of flour and two cups of sugar; it should be one cup of sugar and two cups of flour!

   Response:_____

   _____

7. Your audiogram indicates that you have a hearing loss for high frequency sounds.

   Response:_____

   _____

8. Your appointment with Dr. Pepper is scheduled for next Thursday at 3:00 p.m.

   Response:_____

   _____

9. I was looking at the telephone bill and was relieved to see it was only $16 for last month.

   Response:_____

   _____

10. The weather forecast for this coming weekend calls for rain on Saturday and clearing on Sunday.

    Response:_____

    _____

Answers and Discussion

Any statement that reiterates the main facts of the sentence but uses different phrasing is acceptable. The following are samples of acceptable responses for exercise 6:

1. John's flight to Tucson, Arizona, arrives at 6:40.

2. Cousin Betty had twins on Thursday. Please inform Brian.

3. You got 93 on the mid-term.

4. Harry and I are traveling to Kenya in September.

5. Darrell, Ron, and David made the team.

6. Change the recipe to one cup sugar and two cups flour.

7. A high frequency hearing loss was shown on your audiogram.

8. Next Thursday at 3:00 you will see Dr. Pepper.

9. Whew! Only a $16 telephone bill for July!

10. The weather report says we'll have rain this Saturday and clearing this Sunday.

Exercise 8. Using Expressive Strategies

Here are some more examples of situations where there is a communication breakdown. Use the expressive continuum if you need help. Choose the strategy you think would work best in each of the following situations.

Expressive Communication Breakdown Continuum*

Person you are talking to—

Understood nothing	Understood one key word	Understood more than one key word	Understood almost everything	Understood everything
A	**B**	**C**	**D**	**E**

You—

Repeat slowly	Repeat rest of sentence	Repeat rest of sentence	Repeat rest of sentence	Ask to confirm
Rephrase	Say another key word	Say another key word	Spell missed word	Summarize
Say sentence in blocks	Use gestures	Use gestures		
Say key word	Spell another key word	Spell another key word		
Use shorter phrase	Use shorter phrase			
Spell keyword				
Use gestures				
Write it	Write it	Write it	Write it	Write it

*B. Jarboe, S. Bally 04/84

A. You and your Uncle Bill are discussing plans for a trip to Baltimore to see a baseball game. He says, "OK. I'll pick you up at ____." You can't understand the end of the sentence. You

    1. Give him some paper and a pencil and ask him to write a note.

    2. Tell him to spell the words you missed.

    3. Tell him what you understood and ask him to repeat the rest.

    4. Say, "Huh?"

B. You are in Roy Rogers. It is very crowded. You have ordered a "chicken dinner" three times, but the waitress still doesn't understand you. You

    1. Think of a way to rephrase.

    2. Act like a chicken to give her the idea.

    3. Spell c-h-i-c-k-e-n.

    4. Write "one chicken dinner" on a note and give it to her.

C. You have a severe pain in your abdomen. The doctor has asked you where it hurts. When you reply, "My abdomen," he doesn't understand. You

    1. Say, "Here," and point to the exact spot.

    2. Rephrase and say, "In my tummy."

    3. Walk out to the nurse's desk to get a pencil and paper and write a note.

    4. Spell a-b-d-o-m-e-n.

D. Your friend is telling you about a really great restaurant. As he tells you the name of it, you begin to cough and you miss the name. You look up and

    1. Ask him to repeat it.

    2. Ask him to write it down on a piece of paper.

    3. Nod and pretend you understand when you don't.

    4. Ask him where it is located and see if you can guess the name.

E. You are in a supermarket. The next item on your list is pimentos. You ask the clerk where they are. He doesn't understand. You

    1. Try saying it again.

    2. Rephrase it to, "They look like sliced tomatoes in a glass jar."

    3. Spell p-i-m-e-n-t-o.

    4. Point to the word on your grocery list.

F. You have told your grandfather the name of your fiancé twice before, but he doesn't seem to remember. You repeat the name three times and spell it, but he still doesn't understand. Finally, you

   1. Give up.

   2. Rephrase her name.

   3. Write a note with the name in big letters.

   4. Say it again and again until he understands.

Answers and Discussion

A. 1. This is not the best strategy at this time. You have only missed a small part of the sentence; it's hardly worth it to get out the pencil and paper to write.

2. This might be a good strategy if you only missed one word, but at this point, you're not sure how many words you've missed.

3. This is probably the best strategy. It helps him to know what you did understand and what you didn't understand, and it helps him to focus on repeating only what you didn't understand.

4. This is a dumb way to get a person to repeat something.

B. 1. It would be hard to think of a way to rephrase "chicken dinner," but if you can, more power to you.

2. This might work, but it also might be embarrassing.

3. This might be a good strategy if the restaurant weren't so crowded and people were not waiting behind you in line. Use it another time.

4. This is probably the best strategy. You might write down your order while you're waiting in line if you know they're crowded and the waitress might have difficulty understanding you.

C. 1. This is probably an effective way because you're showing him or her exactly where it hurts.

2. This might be a good way to do it, but pointing to the exact spot is more accurate.

3. This is time consuming and should only be used as a last resort. This is not a bad idea but 1 is probably quicker and more effective.

4. This is a good alternate strategy, but 1 is probably quicker and more effective.

D. 1. This is a good idea. You acknowledge that you understand that he's talking about restaurants; just zero in on the specific name.

2. This may not be necessary and, again, should be used as a last resort. You're probably not in a hurry in this situation.

3. This is a stupid approach; you never learn anything this way.

4. This is rather silly when you can get right to the point.

E. 1. This is not a bad idea, but I think you can find a better one.

2. This would probably be more difficult than the word *pimentos* itself.

3. Spelling it is not bad if you know your speech is good enough for him to understand the spelling.

4. This is probably the best answer. After all, you already have it written down in your grocery list, and all you need to do is point. Besides, the clerk is probably busy.

F. 1. Giving up never solves anything.

2. If you can find a way to rephrase someone's name, I'm going to be really impressed!

---

3. This is probably a good idea in this situation. If it's in big letters, he'll be able to read it easily, and you can give him the piece of paper to help him remember.

4. If you've already repeated again and again and again, this probably won't help more than it already has.

Remember that oftentimes there are several different strategies you can use. Use your logic to decide which one will work best first, second, third, and so forth.

Exercise 9. Using Expressive Repair Strategies

In this exercise, XXX indicates words or phrases that you are unable to understand (through hearing or speechreading) and ??? indicates words or phrases of which you are unsure. In a conversation with a nonsigning individual, one or more of the following strategies may be appropriate for each situation. You may review the explanations of these strategies if you are not sure what they are. In the blank before each situation, write the letter of the appropriate strategy or strategies which you would use.

A. Repetition

B. Clarification or confirmation

C. Rephrasing

D. Spelling

E. Signing or fingerspelling (gesture or mime)

F. Key word

G. Digits

H. Counting

I. Writing

_____ 1. The receptionist at your hearing aid dealer tells you, "Your appointment will be next Thursday at XXX in the afternoon."

_____ 2. The information desk at the telephone company tells you, "Go to see Miss XXX in Room 205 to help you solve your problem with your telephone bill."

_____ 3. You have given the man at the movie theatre the money for your ticket, but he does not give you your ticket for some reason. He says, "XXX XXX XXX."

_____ 4. You have always taken the 5:45 Metroliner to New York. You want to be sure that it is leaving on time. The ticket teller says, "Your train leaves at XXX."

_____ 5. You are reporting for a job interview downtown. The secretary says, "See Mr. Kusovich (???) in Room 114."

_____ 6. You are in a shop and are asking the price of a gold chain. The salesclerk says, "It costs $36.00 plus XXX tax."

_____ 7. You are standing on a street corner as a friend gives you directions to the nearest post office. A truck passes by. You hear your friend say, "The post office XXX XXX XXX left at XXX."

_____ 8. You are looking at some shoes in a store window trying to decide if you should buy them. Your friend say, "Those shoes are really XXX."

_____ 9. You are visiting your friend. Your friend's son asks you, "May I have some XXXs?"

_____ 10. Your uncle is telling you about a fish he caught. He tells you it was bigger than a salami(???).

Answers and Discussion

The appropriate responses for exercise 8 are listed in order of priority. For most situations more than one strategy may work. If you select any of these, you are on the right track!

Responses:

1. C, G, or H	6. A, C, or G
2. A, C, D, or I	7. A
3. A or C	8. C or F
4. B or A	9. B, D, or F
5. A or D	10. B, C, or E

Exercise 10. Using Expressive Repair Strategies

Now try a situation. For each communication breakdown, choose a strategy from the list in the last exercise. Write the letter in the parentheses. Then write your response.

You are at the box office buying a ticket for your favorite hockey team's next game.

Cashier: May I help you?

You: Yes, I'd like to buy four tickets for the game next week.

Cashier: What XXX?

1. You: ( )_____

_____

Cashier: What seXXX?

2. You: ( )_____

_____

Cashier: S-e-c-t-i-o-n

You: Oh! Thank you. I'd like a seat on the west side of the arena.

Cashier: You want the XXX or XXX dollar seats?

3. You: ( )_____

_____

Cashier: 8/9 (???) or $10.00.

4. You: ( )_____

_____

Cashier: E-i-g-h-t

You: I'll take the $8.00 seats. What time does the game start?

Cashier: XXX starts at 7:30. The game starts at 8:00.

5. You: ( )_____

_____

Cashier: There's a warm-up for the team.

6. You: ( )_____

_____

Cashier: You know, practice.

You: Oh, yes. Thanks for your help.

Cashier: Bye.

You: Bye for now.

Answers and Discussion

1. (A) I'm sorry I didn't understand you. Would you please say that again?

2. (D) I still didn't understand. Could you spell that for me? or

   (F) I still didn't understand. Could you give me the second word by itself?

3. (C) What are the prices again?

4. (B) Did you say 8 or 9?

5. (B) or (F) The game starts at 8:00. What happens at 7:30?

6. (C) Something for the team? Could you say that in a different way? or

(F) What is happening with the team?

Now, try setting up your own situations and practice with a friend. Choose situations that have been problematic for you. See how versatile you can be in repairing breakdowns.

Exercise 11. Speaker-Based Problems

Here are some situations involving problems with the speaker. Using the elements of an effective, assertive approach, consider the consequences of your approach and then write what you might say in each example to improve the situation.

1. You and Mary Pat have gone to McDonald's. Mary Pat is telling you about her new baby, but she is eating a Big Mac and speechreading is difficult.

   You say, "_____

   _____."

2. You and Rich are discussing your trip to Miami. Rich is saying something about your route, but the map is in front of his face.

   You say, "_____

   _____."

3. Dr. Lotterperson is discussing your grade with you. His radio is playing and making it difficult to understand his speech.

   You say, "_____

   _____."

4. You met your old friend Mary on the beach at Ocean City. It is difficult to follow the conversation because the sun is shining in your eyes.

   You say, "_____

   _____."

5. Monica is giving you directions to the YWCA. She is going so fast that you can't understand.

   You say, "_____

   _____."

6. You and your friend are in Georgetown. A man in a turban and long robe approaches and asks you a question. You do not understand one word.

You say, "_____

_____."

7. The man at the information booth at the Smithsonian, after noticing your hearing aid, is yelling the time for the movie at you. It sounds very distorted through your hearing aid, and you can't understand.

You say, "_____

_____."

8. You and your friend are at a parade. He is telling you about his vacation while he tries to watch the parade. You get half of each sentence as he looks back and forth.

You say, "_____

_____."

9. Brenda is telling you the latest gossip. She is whispering, and your hearing aid isn't helping you to understand.

You say, "_____

_____."

10. The clerk at Sears has noticed you were signing to your friends and is now telling you about the bicycle you are looking at. However, he is exaggerating his mouth and gesturing wildly. You have no idea what he is saying.

You say, "_____

_____."

Answers and Discussion

The following are examples of appropriate responses. Yours may vary somewhat but should have the same basic components.

1. Gee, Mary Pat, I'm having a tough time speechreading. It would probably be better if we ate first and then talked. I'm really eager to hear about your new baby.

2. Rich, could you please lower the map? Speechreading is difficult, and I don't want to miss your ideas.

3. Would you mind if I turned down your radio, Dr. Lotterperson? I'm having difficulty following this conversation.

4. Let's go up to the boardwalk and sit in the shade with a nice cool drink. This sun is making it really difficult for me to speechread.

5. Monica, could we please go over these directions one step at a time. I don't want to miss anything.

6. I'm sorry I don't understand you clearly enough to help. Perhaps you should try a police officer or shopkeeper.

7. Thanks for speaking up, but with my hearing aid it really isn't necessary. I appreciate your thoughtfulness.

8. Let's watch the parade now and talk about your vacation later. I don't want to miss anything, and this parade is too distracting.

9. Let's go someplace private and talk. Your whispering just isn't loud enough for my hearing aid to pick up, and I don't want to miss a detail!

10. Sir, I'm having difficulty understanding you. If you would just face me and speak naturally it would really help me to understand.

Now try your new strategies for speechreading in some real situations. Remember to anticipate your speechreading needs beforehand, select appropriate strategies, and use them in an effective way. Good luck!

6. Speechreading Tests and Methods

Every person learning speechreading and every teacher teaching speechreading is interested in finding out (1) how good a speechreader the student is naturally, (2) how much improvement a student makes during training, and (3) what the student's specific strengths and weaknesses are. Speechreading tests have been developed to try to provide this information. All speechreading tests, however, have limitations, and it is important for users to understand those weaknesses. It is hoped this chapter will give the reader an understanding of both the strengths and weaknesses of these tools.

It is also useful for the reader to have some knowledge of the various speechreading methods that are used during training. This chapter presents an overview of methods currently used by speechreading teachers and relates those methods to speechreading systems developed at the beginning of the twentieth century. It is believed that this perspective can help the student better use the procedures offered in therapy. Some of the methods described in this chapter are illustrated in chapter 7 with exercises developed by speechreading students.

Reasons for Giving Speechreading Tests

Speechreading tests are used to measure the basic speechreading ability of a person to determine whether he or she is a good, fair, or poor speechreader. An individual, however, can perform well on one test of speechreading and poorly on another simply because one test is easier than the other. Which test measures the person's true speechreading skills? For example, Mr. Jones may score 90% on Test A but only 40% on Test B. Is he an excellent or a poor speechreader? Unfortunately no one knows which of the many

measurement tools on the market best evaluates what a speechreader must do in daily life. When someone is described as a good or a poor speechreader, it usually means he or she has done well on a particular test. The person may or may not be communicating well in daily life. Successful functioning in life activities may involve not only speechreading of sentences but also use of residual hearing and communication strategies. Therefore, one must be more specific in defining what is meant by being a good speechreader.

When a person is considered a good speechreader, it is important to ask, "Compared to whom?" Does it mean that he or she understands speech better than most hearing adults, most hearing-impaired adults, or most adults in general? Perhaps the individual is being compared only to the other members of a class. In order to properly interpret results of a speechreading test, one must know the population to whom the person is being compared.

A second use of speechreading tests is to evaluate progress in therapy. A student is given a speechreading test at the beginning of training and a comparable one at the end to see how much improvement has occurred. These tests, which are usually lists of unrelated sentences, evaluate how much improvement a person has made in the ability to speechread sentences. There is no assurance, however, that this kind of improvement indicates better understanding of conversation in everyday life situations. This lack of *validity* is one of the major problems with speechreading tests. A third use of speechreading tests is for proper placement of students within a training program. In order to prepare lessons that provide the right amount of challenge it is necessary to group students with similar skills. Otherwise, a lesson may be too difficult for some and too easy for others. Although teachers can compensate to some degree for differences in skill level by varying the amount of voice or the number of clues used when presenting material, teaching is much more effective if the students' skills do not vary too much. A speechreading test given to all individuals in a class allows the teacher to form appropriate groups.

In the ideal situation, speechreading students are grouped for instruction with others at the same skill level. Most teaching situations, however, are not ideal. The teacher is required to instruct people have widely different levels of skill. To ensure that everyone experiences the right amount of challenge, the teacher must use different amounts of voice and different ways of presenting material. For example, Mrs. A is an average speechreader while Mr. G has excellent skills. Mrs. A might be seated directly in front of the teacher so that the teacher's face is always clearly visible. Mr. G, on the other hand, might be seated to the side of the teacher to make speechreading more challenging. Speechreading tests provide the information needed to determine who needs more and who needs less challenge in a group.

A fourth use of speechreading tests is to help the teacher decide which teaching methods are most useful for a given student. The earlier chapters talked about the need to visually recognize sounds, as well as the importance of using context and situational clues. Some people do well at recognizing visible sounds on the lips but have a great deal of difficulty using context and situational information. Others can use the redundancies of language well but do not easily differentiate between sounds which are recognizable on the lips. Obviously, different training procedures are needed for the two types of individuals. Some speechreading tests evaluate specific sound recognition and others look at a person's ability to use context. In a teaching environment, tests are used diagnostically in this way to help the therapist plan appropriate therapy.

A fifth use of speechreading tests is to define how much speechreading is contributing to a person's overall communication. To do this, three comparable forms of the same test might be used: one form is administered with sound only, a second with speechreading only, and a third uses both speechreading and listening. This type of evaluation can yield valuable information about the way a person functions. It can demonstrate how much a properly fitted hearing aid used with speechreading can help understanding of connected speech. For some people, improvement of speechreading is the major reason for using a hearing aid. If sound is not helpful to speechreading, that needs to be known. We have found that for most people, aided hearing and speechreading together work better than either one alone.

Finally, speechreading tests can be used to find out which speakers are easiest to understand. Ask a group of people to speechread several individuals delivering similar material and compare the scores for the different speakers. The speaker receiving the highest score is considered the most understandable. This use of speechreading tests is important for research and for selection of speakers in the preparation of new test materials.

Problems with Speechreading Tests

A good speechreading test is supposed to evaluate how a person speechreads in real life situations. We do not know, however, what kind of material is most appropriate. Most speechreading tests consist of lists of unrelated sentences containing everyday language. Is such material typical of normal conversation? If an individual performs poorly on such a test, does it mean he or she is a poor speechreader in a conversational situation? In actual conversation one sentence logically follows another. The speechreader has the benefit of contextual clues, but such clues are not present on a test using unrelated sentences.

Perhaps the vocabulary on the test is not appropriate. If the vocabulary and sentence structure are too difficult or unfamiliar, the person may do poorly even though in actual life situations he or she may function quite well. Although most of the sentence tests designed for adults use vocabulary that is comparable to a third-grade reading level, they still are not suitable for people who are unfamiliar with English idioms or some types of English sentence structures. Unless the vocabulary and sentence structure are familiar to the person, the test is really not evaluating speechreading skill; it is evaluating language or educational level. On the other hand, if the language is too easy, the test will not differentiate between skilled and less skilled speechreaders. Everyone will perform well.

Sentence tests are usually scored by giving the speechreader credit for every word, or with some tests every important word, identified correctly. In real life, however, it is not necessary for a speechreader to understand every word a speaker uses, only enough of the words to grasp the meaning. A literal repetition task not only deviates from real life requirements, but also may evaluate the speechreader's memory rather than speechreading skills.

Perhaps the best kind of test involves the ability to understand stories. What kind of stories should be used, however? Should teachers use jokes, stories about famous people, conversations, etc.? What topics and vocabulary would be universally acceptable? What kind of material best evaluates what the speechreader must do every day? We don't have good answers to these questions.

It is more difficult to score story tests. With this kind of procedure, it is necessary to determine whether the person understands the meaning of the story. The most obvious way to do that is to present questions which the person must answer correctly. It is necessary, however, to decide what makes an answer correct or if an answer can be partially correct. Different examiners may not score a question/answer test the same way.

Another problem relates to the kind of speaker used for the speechreading test. Everyone, particularly the hearing-impaired person, is aware that some people are easier to speechread than others. Is it more appropriate to use a speaker who is clearly understood for a speechreading test or a person who is more difficult to understand? In real life situations, people must communicate with both types of speakers. Which test gives a more realistic approximation of the skill of the speechreader? Is it better to use a male speaker, a female, an elderly person, or a child? Perhaps several speakers should be used in a speechreading test. A speechreader will perform very differently when the same test materials are presented by different speakers. Which type of speaker best represents speechreading requirements of everyday conversation?

Similarly, it is not known which environmental conditions provide the most valid approximation of everyday speechreading demands. All speechreading tests use full-face presentation. Is this desirable? People are often required to speechread from the side. During tests, lighting and distance factors are controlled to make speechreading conditions optimal. Is this procedure most representative of real life speechreading? There are no good answers to these questions.

What Should an Ideal Test Be Like?

Berger (1972) discusses the factors that should be considered in constructing such a tool. Following is a summary of some of his ideas.

1. The test should be valid. It should parallel the kind of conversation a person encounters in daily life.

2. It should be appropriate for the specific population it is to be used with. This means that vocabulary and sentence structure should be selected so that the test items are measuring

speechreading and not the language or educational level of the individual.

3. Speakers should be selected carefully. In an ideal test, there should be a range of speakers varying in speechreading clarity. In less than ideal conditions, it is generally best to settle for a speaker who is easy to speechread.

4. The difficulty of the test items should be considered. They should neither be so difficult that all testees miss them nor so easy that everyone obtains a high score.

5. Under ideal conditions there should be a range of test conditions varying from optimal in all respects to very difficult. Since this is not practical, test conditions should be carefully controlled. The speaker should be clearly visible. Lighting and distance conditions should be favorable to the speechreader. The items should be presented at a comfortable rate, and all examinees should be able to view the speaker at no greater than a forty-five degree angle.

The ideal or perfect test does not exist and perhaps never will. Because tests vary in many ways, there is no absolute measure of speechreading. A person may score high on one test and low on another. Therefore, whenever someone's speechreading skills are described these considerations must be kept in mind.

Most Commonly Used Speechreading Tests

There are many speechreading tests available today. Some use words; some use sentences; a few use stories. Some are on film or videotape; others are live-voice tests. It is also possible to assess speechreading ability informally. For a more complete discussion of the speechreading tests available on the market, see chapter 8 in Berger (1972), chapter 4 in O'Neill and Oyer (1981), and chapter 7 in Jeffers and Barley (1971).

Informal Assessment

There are times when judgments of speechreading skill are made by observing how well a person understands speech, using only or primarily visual cues. Teachers often assess hearing-impaired children's speechreading skills by observing which children are the best speechreaders.

In addition audiologists, during an initial session with a hearing-impaired client, sometimes attempt to discover how much that person depends on speechreading. The audiologist may lower the level of his or her voice or unobtrusively cover the mouth while speaking. The client who depends heavily on speechreading will not be overly disturbed by the first maneuver but may be considerably upset by the second. Sometimes, it is obvious that a person is visually attentive. Such an individual carefully watches every movement of the speaker's lips.

Informal methods are used in testing young children. The examiner plays games in which the child must follow commands or identify pictures or objects. Obviously the vocabulary must be carefully selected.

Reliability or repeatability is an important concern with informal testing because it is impossible to exactly duplicate the same testing conditions or manner of presentation. In situations, however, where a general impression is needed or where formal tests are not possible, informal evaluation can be very valuable.

Formal Tests

Although there are tests available that use nonsense syllables, words, and stories as stimuli, the most commonly used tests for adults consist of lists of unrelated sentences. These tests use vocabulary that is comparable to a third-grade reading level and can be used with older children as well as adults. The sentences use everyday language that is familiar. Within each list, sentence length varies from two to perhaps ten words. Each test has several forms which have been found equivalent in speechreading difficulty. It is possible to use one test list for pretherapy evaluation and another for posttherapy evaluation. Research has also indicated that various sentence tests agree well with each other provided they are presented by the same speaker under the same conditions. Therefore, lists may be used interchangeably if presentation constraints are kept in mind.

The speaker says each sentence once or twice, and the speechreader must write every word recognized. Some tests are scored by giving one point for each correct word while other tests give one point for each key (important) word identified correctly.

The major problem with the sentence tests relates to validity. Even though the sentences represent everyday American speech, the sentences on the list are not related to each other. This is not typical of conversation where one sentence follows another logically and the speechreader can get important clues to meaning from the context. It is legitimate to ask whether such a test evaluates what a person must do to handle conversation.

The Binnie Test (Binnie, Montgomery, & Jackson, 1974) is very different from the sentence tests. It uses nonsense syllables such as /pa/, /fa/, /la/ instead of sentences. The student is given an answer sheet with twenty nonsense syllables written across the top. For each of the 100 items in the test, the speaker says a nonsense syllable in the following way: "I will say (nonsense syllable)." The student then puts a mark under the nonsense syllable he or she thinks is correct.

The purpose of the test is to find out whether the student can identify those consonants which are visible. An item is considered correct if the student's response falls into the correct consonant homophene group. For example, if the speaker said the nonsense syllable /pa/ and the student identified it as /ba/, that is considered correct. It is not possible to see the difference between /pa/ and /ba/. If the student chooses /fa/, that is considered an error because it is possible to see the difference between /pa/ and /fa/. The clinician does not use this test to evaluate overall speechreading skill but to find out what a student needs to work on. If a student gets a high score on the Binnie Test, that means he or she is already identifying all possible visual differences between consonants. Training in visual discrimination is not necessary. However, other tests may show that the student needs a great deal of work to better use context clues.

Speechreading Tests and Communication Function

A number of communication or hearing handicap scales have been developed to determine the real-life communication function of hearing-impaired adults. A good discussion of these scales can be found in chapters 2 and 6 of Alpiner (1982). One of these scales is the Denver Scale of Communication Function (Alpiner, Chevrette, Glascoe, Metz, & Olsen, 1982) that evaluates a person's perceived communication difficulty and anxiety as it relates to communication. Olsen, Alpiner, Chevrette, Glascoe, and Metz (1972) gave the Denver Scale to a group of twenty-five hearing-impaired adults before and after a ten-week rehabilitation program. They also administered a videotaped speechreading test. They found that after ten weeks of therapy there were reported improvements in communication function and reductions in anxiety as measured by the Denver Scale. Speechreading scores, however, did not show the same improvement. Undoubtedly, many other clinicians have found similar results with clients. Apparently, it is possible to improve ability to speechread sentences but still not improve overall communication function. The reverse is also quite likely. It is important to remember this limitation of speechreading tests when interpreting scores.

Speechreading Methods

All of the speechreading methods used today are modifications of procedures from one of the four older systems developed during the early twentieth century. Two of the four systems are considered primarily **analytic** because they focus on visual recognition of sounds as they appear on the lips. The other two systems are considered primarily **synthetic** because they emphasize mind training, the ability of the speechreader to use context to understand the meaning of what is said. These systems will be described briefly because every speechreading teacher uses some combination or modification of some of these procedures.

The Early Speechreading Systems

Primarily Analytic Systems

Jena and Mueller-Walle. The Jena Method was brought to America from Germany by Anna Bunger (Bunger, 1952). According to this method, the speechreader learns all of the sound movements by imitating everything the speaker says. The theory is that after enough training in imitation, the speechreader should be able to remember the feel of the sounds as he or she watches a speaker. This is called kinesthetic awareness and is supposed to substitute for hearing. The speechreader who has developed kinesthetic awareness should be able to more easily understand others. We have no evidence to prove or disprove this theory, but some modern speechreading teachers still use imitation of speech in their programs.

The basis of the Jena system is the syllable drill. At the beginning of each lesson a sound movement is introduced. After the sound movement is learned, there is drill on repetition of syllables containing the sound. The next step is drill on words made from the syllables and finally on sentences containing those words. The sentences can lead to a story that is followed by questions prob-

ing understanding of its meaning. The rhythms of speech are considered important. Therefore, when students imitate syllable drills, they do so using different rhythmic patterns.

Although exercises on stories are related to meaning, the Jena Method is considered primarily an analytic method because the basic goal of therapy is training the eye to recognize the sounds of speech. Therefore, story material is not always relevant or meaningful.

The Mueller-Walle Method was introduced to America in 1902 by Martha Bruhn (Bruhn, 1949) who learned it from Mueller-Walle in Germany. Like Jena, it is primarily analytical and is also based on the syllable drill. It does, however, have more synthetic components than the Jena Method.

One exercise used by many teachers today is called *add-a-word* or *add-a-phrase*. Words and sentences are developed from the syllable drills. Then the first part of the sentence is repeated, but new words or phrases are added to make new sentences. A common way to use this technique is for practice of expressions that are used frequently. For example, if a student needs practice on question words, the teacher might develop an exercise such as the following:

> "Where are you going?"
> "Where do you live?"
> "Where do you work?"

Other exercises introduced by Mueller-Walle include

1. Work on homophenes. The students identify a group of homophenous words and select the correct word from information provided by a sentence.

2. Exercise story. The teacher introduces a story to the group by using full voice to teach important vocabulary. In addition, she or he presents a group of sentences about the story (clue

sentences). The story is then presented using reduced voice and questions are asked.

Primarily Synthetic Methods

Nitchie (1950) **and Kinzie** (1931, 1936). Nitchie and Kinzie believed that both the eye and the mind must be trained but that mind training was more important. Although there are both analytic and synthetic components in their methods, the emphasis is on the synthetic approach. Words, not syllables, are used for eye training. During a typical lesson a sound movement is explained. The students then speechread practice words containing that sound movement, followed by sentences using the practice words.

The basic difference between the Kinzie and Nitchie methods is that the former presents all materials except instructions without voice. All other speechreading systems use reduced voice in presenting material to hard-of-hearing students and full voice with severely and profoundly hearing-impaired individuals. The Kinzies also developed graded speechreading material for children. In all other respects the Nitchie and Kinzie systems were similar and are discussed together.

An exercise used in every lesson is called *contrast words*. A word containing the sound introduced in the lesson is paired with another word containing a sound taught in a previous lesson. The student learns to differentiate between the two sound movements by watching them on the speaker's lips. The contrast word exercise has been adapted by more recent speechreading teachers such as Jeffers, whose speechreading system will be discussed later in this chapter.

Following is an example of a Nitchie Method lesson.

Sound: /p, b, m/ The lips are shut.

Explanation: For /p/ as in *pie*, /b/ as in *by*, and /m/ as in *my*, the lips open from a closed position. All three sounds look the same.

Practice Words: meet, patch, pound
bell, moon, paid
ball, book, boat

Contrast Words: pet-peat-feet-heap-heat
beet-veet-eeb-eve
met-vet-team-teave

Sentences: Where shall **I meet** you for lunch?
We **meet** every day during the week.
I thought I heard the **bell** ring.
There is a **ball** game at the stadium today.

Notice that some of the contrast items are not meaningful words. Also the sentences are not related to each other, and the practice words don't always give useful clues to the meaning of the sentences. Although these sentences are less analytic than those used by the Jena or Mueller-Walle methods, they are not the best kind of synthetic training because there are very few clues available from context.

Other synthetic exercises include:

1. Homophene exercises. Homophenous words are identified and recognized from the context of sentences.

2. Work on idioms. The meanings of specific idiomatic expressions are explained. The students practice speechreading the idioms in sentences.

3. Short stories followed by questions.

More Recent Speechreading Methods

All of the more recent speechreading methods are modifications of the four older systems—Jena, Mueller-Walle, Nitchie, and Kinzie. In general, the emphasis of the more recent methods is on synthetic activities.

Morkovin-Moore Training Films. The Morkovin-Moore training films (Morkovin & Moore, 1948) use conversations that might occur in actual life situations. Titles of some of the films are *The Family Dinner, At the Bank, At the Grocery Store,* and *At the Service Station.* Other films are based on the interests of children such as *The Cowboy, Barbara's New Shoes*, and *Magic*.

Although the concept of using life situations for speechreading training is excellent, the films are not widely used because they are old and technically poor. The people on the films are not easy to speechread, and some of the scenes do not seem natural. The situational clues which are supposed to help the speechreader understand the dialogue actually are of little value. Nevertheless, the concept of role-playing life situations to teach speechreading is used extensively by speechreading teachers using live voice.

Jeffers Method. The speechreading method described by Jeffers and Barley (1971) is based on the concept that speechreading requires training in three areas:

1. The ability to recognize visible sounds quickly and accurately.

2. The ability to use all contextual, situational, and nonverbal clues available to correctly fill in the speech that the eye cannot see.

3. The ability to be flexible, to quickly change one's mind about what was seen if the original idea doesn't make sense as the conversation continues.

The specific exercises used in this approach have been taken directly from earlier methods or are modifications of earlier procedures. The Jeffers and Barley system allows the teacher to use any technique that meets the needs of the group.

The procedure for developing visual sound recognition is called the *quick recognition exercise* and is a modification of Nitchie's contrast words. The teacher shows three words that are the same except for one sound, e.g., *might, fight, right*. The three words are spoken in different orders, and the students must repeat the words in correct sequence. The teacher may vary the speed and rhythm as the words are spoken.

Many different types of exercises are used to develop flexibility and ability to use contextual and

situational redundancy, including the following:

1. Quick Identification Exercises on homophenes. The teacher says a word and asks the student to identify it as well as other words which look the same. After several homophenes have been identified, the teacher speaks sentences containing the homophenes. The student must recognize the correct homophene by using the context of the sentence.

2. Familiar sentences on a single theme. The student is told the topic, and the teacher speaks sentences or questions about that topic. The student responds by repeating enough of the sentence to indicate understanding of the meaning. He or she may also write the sentence, answer a question, or comment on a statement. The sentences may relate to an important life situation, to a student's major field, to language used socially on a job, to language used during a job interview, or anything else of significance to the student.

3. Drill on familiar words and phrases (e.g., days of the week, numbers, or question words). The add-a-phrase technique from Mueller-Walle is sometimes used for this type of work.

4. Unrelated sentences. The student must identify sentences that cannot be predicted from the situation or the preceding sentence. Usually a clue word is given unless the speechreader is very proficient. Speechreading unrelated sentences is difficult because the student lacks situational or contextual clues to help understanding. This kind of practice is useful, however, for dealing with sudden changes of topic.

5. Stories. Stories can vary in length and complexity to suit the speechreading proficiency of the student. A story exercise can be performed in several different ways.

   a. The teacher may read the story and ask the student to identify the topic.

   b. The teacher may reveal the topic and provide a number of clue sentences that give information about the story. Then she or he tells the story and asks questions about it.

c. The teacher may drill on vocabulary used in the story, then tell the story and ask questions.

d. The student may identify each sentence individually after which the teacher presents the entire story for meaning.

6. Quizzes, Riddles, or Games. Crossword puzzles may be adapted for speechreading practice. Team competition among two groups in a speechreading class can enliven a lesson. The speechreading exercises in chapter 7 contain many examples of such activities.

7. Skits and Conversations. The teacher and a helper or two students may present a dialogue about some real life situation. The others must correctly answer questions or perform activities indicating understanding. This type of exercise is handled in much the same way as the Morkovin-Moore films.

Other Synthetic Exercises. Raymond Hull (1976) has developed some exercises that train the speechreader to use the linguistic redundancy of language. He believes that speechreading is a purely synthetic skill and that skill development should be based entirely on mind training. Following are descriptions of several of his procedures.

1. Right and Wrong Information. The teacher first writes a sentence on the board and then speaks a sentence that may be the same or different. The student must decide whether the two sentences are the same or different and, if different, in what way. For example, the sentence on the board might be, *Where* are you going? The spoken sentence might be, *When* are you going?

2. Filling in the Gaps. The teacher writes a sentence on the board but leaves out key words or phrases. She or he then speaks the sentence and the student must identify the missing words. For example,

Written sentence: What _____ is _____ today?

Spoken sentence: What time is dinner today?

3. Structure of the Language. This procedure is similar to filling in the gaps. The teacher writes a sentence on the board with all words missing except one. Then the sentence is spoken. If the student cannot identify it, another word is added, and the sentence is spoken again. Words are continually added until the sentence is understood. For example,

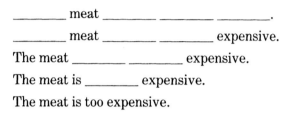

_____ meat _____ _____ _____.

_____ meat _____ _____ expensive.

The meat _____ _____ expensive.

The meat is _____ expensive.

The meat is too expensive.

4. How Would You Say It? How Would the Listener Say It? The teacher identifies a situation such as going to the doctor. The students are asked to suggest sentences that people might say in that situation. The class practices speechreading the sentences.

Cued Speech

In chapter 3 two major problems of speechreading discussed were that (1) many of the sounds of English are not visible on the lips, and (2) many sounds look identical or similar on the lips. Therefore, a skilled speechreader must rely heavily on the use of language context. The orally educated, prelingually deaf child must learn language largely through speechreading and whatever residual hearing is available. Because speechreading is highly dependent on knowledge of language, the prelingually deaf child is faced with a significant problem.

The postlingually hearing-impaired adult who has developed a mental language model can more easily fill in what the eye cannot see. Still, many hearing-impaired adults find it difficult to develop the skill of educated guessing. Their speechreading skills are limited by the problems of visibility and homopheneity.

If all syllables of spoken language could be made to look different on the lips, speech could become totally clear to the eye. Then the deaf child could learn language by watching the lips in much the same way a hearing child learns language through audition. The hearing-impaired adult could rely more on visual sound recognition and less on educated guessing. The problems of homopheneity would not exist.

Cued Speech is an attempt to make all of the syllables of spoken English visually distinctive. It combines information received from lip movements with eight configurations and four positions of one hand. Sounds that look alike or similar on the lips look different on the hands, while sounds that use similar hand movements look different on the lips. The four hand positions cue different groups of vowels. For example, the vowel /ee/ as in *see* is cued at the mouth; the vowel /i/ as in *sit*, which looks similar to /ee/, is cued at the throat. With both lip movements and manual cues, the two vowels are visually distinctive. Consonants are cued using different hand configurations, with homophenous consonants having different hand shapes. For example, /m/ is cued with an open hand, /b/ with four extended fingers, and /p/ with one extended finger. The cues supplied by the hands alone do not allow a person to understand speech; the cues must be used with information from the lips. Below are charts showing the hand positions and configurations for the various sounds of English speech.

The Cued Speech system was developed by Dr. Orin Cornett at Gallaudet College in 1966. Since that time, it has been successfully used by many prelingually deaf children as a method of language development. There is also some indication that the use of Cued Speech improves speechreading even when the manual cues are not used. At present Cued Speech is being tried by small groups of hard-of-hearing adults to facilitate speechreading. For further discussion of Cued Speech see Cornett (1967, 1972).

CUED SPEECH (English)

Chart I: Cues for Vowel Sounds

	Side	Throat	Chin	Mouth
open	ah (father) (got)	a (that)	aw (dog)	
flattened/ relaxed	u (but)	i (is)	e (get)	ee (see)
rounded	oe (home)	oo (book)	ue (blue)	ur (her)

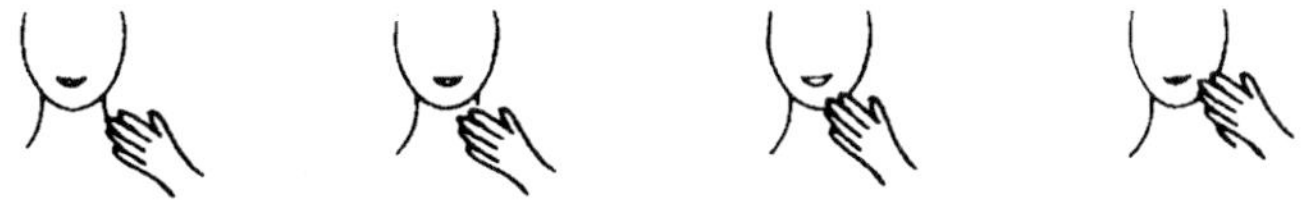

Chart II: Diphthongs

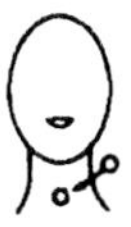

ie (my) 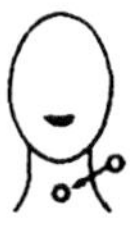   ou (cow) 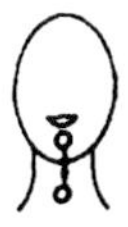   ae (pay) 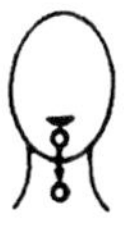   oi (boy)

Chart III: Cues for Consonant Sounds

t,m,f	h,s,r	d,p,zh	ng,y,ch	l,sh,w	k,v,th,z	b,n,wh	g,j,th

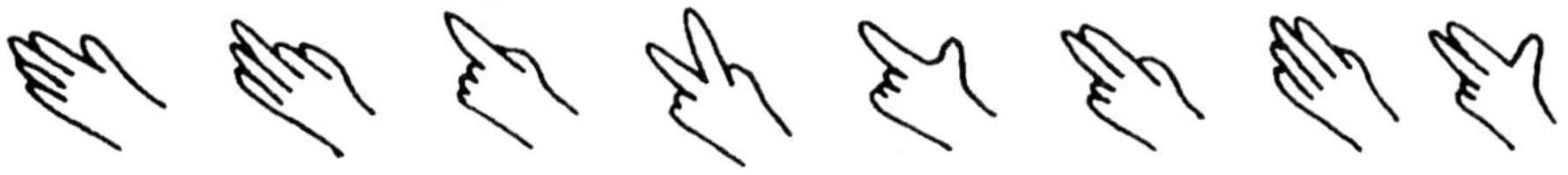

Summary

Speechreading tests are used for a variety of purposes: to assess an individual's speechreading ability, to evaluate progress in therapy, to group students according to level of skill, to determine the contribution of speechreading to a person's overall communication skills, and to decide which speakers are most speechreadable. The validity of all of our existing tests is questionable; none have demonstrated the ability to evaluate the kind of speechreading required in everyday life. Although speechreading tests have their uses, readers must be careful to interpret results with test limitations in mind.

Interest in the use of speechreading for hearing-impaired adults developed at the beginning of the twentieth century. Most of our current methods have been taken from four speechreading systems introduced then.

There are many different procedures and exercises used to teach speechreading. Some are analytical, stressing sound recognition on the lips, and others are synthetic, focusing on use of language and situational redundancy. The teacher chooses those methods and materials which are best for his or her students.

Most teachers use some voice in presenting materials so that students are aware the teacher is speaking but are not able to understand the message only by listening. In addition, most teachers use language in speechreading exercises that is meaningful and useful to the students.

Cued Speech is a system that uses hand cues to supplement what is seen on the lips. It was designed to facilitate language development in young deaf children by making all the syllables of English speech clearly visible and distinctive. Cued Speech has been found to be highly readable by those who know the system. Most children who have been consistently exposed to it at home and in school seem to have done well in their language development. More research is needed.

7. Speechreading Exercises

Introduction

There are several approaches one can use to improve speechreading skills. The best way is to sign up for an individual or group class taught by a speech pathologist, audiologist, or other qualified professional. Such classes may be offered by community speech and hearing centers, hospital or university clinics, and sometimes through adult education programs. Check with your local or state speech and hearing association or the yellow pages of the phone book for sources.

Sometimes, however, such sources are unavailable. The suggestions and exercises in this chapter are for individuals who wish to do some speechreading practice on their own because classes are not available or because they wish to supplement classroom instruction, perhaps in preparation for a specific event. Of course, an individual must ask a member of his or her family, a friend, or someone for assistance. This person must be willing to assume the role of the instructor by speaking the necessary words or sentences in the exercises for the individual to practice speechreading. Answers are given at the end of each exercise.

The following suggestions may be helpful in dealing with problems of homopheneity and improving ability to use context.

Homopheneity

You can increase your ability to speechread words by learning to recognize sounds and their viseme counterparts. For a description of which sounds look alike, see the viseme groupings in chapter 3. Once you have committed these groups to memory it is fairly easy to predict words that may be confused because of homopheneity. Following is one method of determining which words look alike.

Use the word *nine* as an example. First, break the word into its parts.

Nine = /n/ + /i/ + /n/; (/e/) is silent.

Next, think of the sounds that are in the /n/ viseme group: /n/, /t/, /d/. Write these sounds in the following formula:

$$\begin{matrix} n & & & & n \\ t & + & i & + & t & = \\ d & & & & d \end{matrix}$$

The possible words that can occur by combining these sounds are nine, night, dine, died, tine (of a fork), tide, tied, tight. Notice that many words are not spelled the way they sound. So, using this formula, you have discovered eight words that are homophenes. It is necessary to depend on context to determine which of these words is being used in a specific sentence.

Now try the word *fine*.

$$\text{fine} = \begin{matrix} f \\ v \end{matrix} + i + \begin{matrix} n \\ d \end{matrix}$$

The following words are possible: fine, fight, vine, vied.

The ability to speechread by analyzing or recognizing sounds on the lips is most helpful in situations where language is limited to short phrases or single words, such as when a specific question is asked. The question itself limits the context and helps you decide if what you are thinking you see is appropriate. The homophene formula, however, can be used in any situation.

The formula may be used to generate groups of homophenous words for speechreading practice. The words are then put into sentences which provide context, and the sentences are used for practice. For example, each of the homophenes for *fine* can be placed in one or more sentences which are spoken by a friend. Your job is to identify the correct homophene in each sentence. The more homophenes you know, the quicker you can figure out what a speaker is saying. The formula may also be used for speechreading real life situations any time you encounter a word that does not fit the context of the situation.

Words generated through use of the formula can be easily adapted to exercises of your own. Use the exercises in this section under the headings *Homopheniety* and *Phoneme and Specific Word Identification* as models. Select sentences and situations which may be helpful to you in your everyday communication.

Remember, it is a combination of skills and strategies in the use of both hearing and speechreading that makes you a better communicator.

Using Context

The easiest way to create lessons for practicing the use of context is to select a difficult communication situation that you encounter now or have encountered in the past. *Going to the dentist* may be used as an example. Use the model in chapter 5, p. 55, labelled Anticipatory Strategies, Exercise 1, Language I, and the constellation diagram on p. 57 to help you organize your thinking.

First, think about the reason for being in the situation, the people involved, and the physical environment. Consider who begins the communication and in what manner. Do *you* begin by asking the dentist a series of questions or by giving a series of directions? Perhaps the *dentist* begins by asking a series of questions. The language will be different. Your reason for being there (emergency, annual checkup, etc.) and your particular relationship with the dentist (old friend or new dentist) will also influence the kind of language used.

Next anticipate the vocabulary that might occur in the situation. Some of the words might be

Dr. States (name of dentist), appointment, checkup, brush and floss, X rays, cavity, novocaine, drill, and filling. After you have thought of the words, try to predict phrases and sentences that might be used in the situation. Following are some examples using the anticipated vocabulary:

> Good morning, I'm Dr. States.
>
> Make an appointment for a checkup in six months.
>
> Do you brush and floss after every meal?
>
> Your X rays show a cavity in an upper left molar.
>
> Dr. States will be with you in a few minutes.
>
> The filling takes three hours to set so eat only soft foods until then.
>
> I won't start to drill until the novocaine takes effect.

Once you have done this homework, it is worthwhile to practice speechreading the anticipated words, phrases, and sentences with a friend or family member. Finally rehearse the situation by role playing it. When you role play a situation, you pretend to be the people involved and communicate as they would in that situation. Play each role separately. In the situation related to the dentist, you would practice as the dentist, the receptionist, and the patient. By doing this, you become aware of vocabulary and language you hadn't expected.

A dialogue in the dentist's office might go like this:

> Receptionist: Good morning, do you have an appointment?
>
> Patient: Yes, I am (your name) and I have an appointment with Dr. States.
>
> Receptionist: He's still with another patient, but if you have a seat, he'll be ready for you in a few minutes.
>
> Patient: That's fine; please wave to me when he's ready. I am deaf and may not hear you call me.

Receptionist: Yes, I will. When were you here
last? I do not have a record
for you.

Patient: I recently moved here. My hometown
dentist will send the records soon.

Receptionist: I'll need to ask you some
information for our records. . . .

For further practice substitute other situations or
use exercises in this section as models. In the
Games and Quizzes part of this chapter, exercises
entitled U.S. History and Geography, page 123,
and More U.S. History and Geography, Page 124,
are good topical models. The stories and questions
format in the Paragraphs and Related Sentences
exercises is equally good and can be readily
adapted to almost any subject.

Substitute topics, vocabulary, and language that
are relevant to you for your daily lifestyle. Now
try some of the exercises in this chapter.

I. Homopheneity Exercises

As has already been mentioned in chapter 3, homopheneity presents tremendous obstacles to effective speechreading and requires that the speechreader utilize his or her intuitive and synthetic powers to the utmost. Sometimes homophenous words sound different, enabling the speechreader with sufficient hearing to identify the correct word by hearing the difference. Other words, however, not only look the same but also sound the same. Such words are both homophenes (look alike) and homophones (sound alike). The speechreader can rely only on context to correctly identify these words. Exercises in this section provide practice in dealing with both kinds of problems.

Exercises: 1. **Homophenous and Homophonous Words—Animals** by Char Laba

2. **Homophenous Word Practice** by Dan Gunther

3. **Homophene Crossword Puzzle** by Elisca Woodard

4. **Weather Report** by Gail Ploman

Exercise 1. Homophenous and Homophonous Words—Animals

Purpose: To provide practice in developing awareness of homophenous words. These words not only look alike but also sound alike. Therefore, the speechreader must use context to tell the difference.

Materials: paper/pen
sentences

Procedure: Students are to speechread each sentence as the instructor says it and then write a word that sounds and looks the same as the last word in the sentence. Hint: All answers relate to animals.

Sentences: 1. The baby let out a hearty wail.

2. The rotting eggs smelled foul.

3. That last class was such a bore.

4. My sister just had a baby and now I am an aunt.

5. We cheered so loudly our voices became hoarse.

6. Have you seen the movie *Hair?*

7. The bread was made with yeast dough.

8. Old Mother Hubbard's cupboard was bare.

9. The twins are so dear.

Answers: 1. whale; 2. fowl; 3. boar; 4. ant; 5. horse; 6. hare; 7. doe;
8. bear; 9. deer

Exercise 2. Homophenous Word Practice

Purpose: To provide practice in recognizing homophenous words.

Materials: word and answer lists

Procedure: Students are to circle the word in the answer list that is homophenous to the word said by the instructor.

Word List	Answer List			
1. rise	1. pies	mine	rice	lice
2. merge	2. lunch	perch	worst	burn
3. chirp	3. germ	firm	sip	term
4. shows	4. chose	woes	sews	mows
5. beep	5. seep	peep	weep	keep
6. jeep	6. skirt	burp	sheep	churn
7. van	7. fat	cat	rat	ran
8. bird	8. word	pearl	burn	boot
9. mount	9. bound	louse	gout	south
10. fight	10. feud	fend	find	found

Answers: 1. rice; 2. perch; 3. germ; 4. chose; 5. peep; 6. sheep; 7. fat; 8. burn; 9. bound; 10. find

Exercise 3. Homophene Crossword Puzzle

Purpose: To identify homophenous words in sentences to be placed in a crossword puzzle.

Materials: blank crossword puzzle
word list (may be written on a chalkboard or flip chart)

Procedure: If needed, practice speechreading the vocabulary prior to doing the puzzle. Write the homophenous words on the board or chart. The teacher says each sentence, the student identifies the appropriate homophene, and writes it in the crossword puzzle.

Word List: deep, keep, seam, seem, steam, team, Teem

Sentences:

DOWN

1. They _____ to be having trouble with the car.

2. We will watch the football _____ play.

3. Mother sewed up the _____ in my dress.

4. The river is very _____.

ACROSS

1. I bought a new _____ iron.

2. I like to drink _____.

5. Can you _____ a secret?

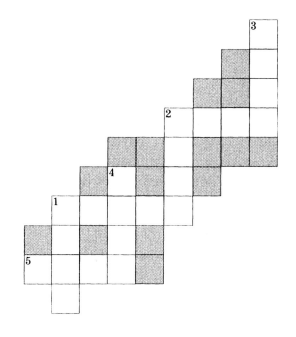

Answers: DOWN 1. seem; 2. team; 3. seam; 4. deep

ACROSS 1. steam; 2. Teem; 3. keep

Exercise 4. Weather Report

Purpose: To provide practice in speechreading numbers that look alike on the lips.

Materials: list of look-alike numbers
weather report
questions

Procedure: A weather report will be read to the students using homophenous numbers. Students are to answer questions about the weather report. They will be asked to identify the clue words in the weather report that enabled them to select the correct number(s).

Look-alike Numbers: 17–70; 15–50; 13–30

Weather Report: Showers and cloudiness this morning. The high temperatures for today will be 70 to 77; low temperatures for tonight will be in the 40s. Tomorrow, partly cloudy with a 15 percent chance of rain that will increase to 50 percent by evening. Tomorrow night, record low of 13 to 15 degrees with high winds.

Questions: 1. What was today's temperature?

2. What temperature is forecast for tonight?

3. What percent chance of rain is forecast for tomorrow?

4. What percent chance of rain is forecast for tomorrow night?

5. Will the temperature tomorrow night be 30 or 13 degrees?

Answers and Discussion

1. 70 to 77—Number 17 looks like 70, but it doesn't make sense to talk about high temperatures of 17 to 77.

2. in the 40s—If we talk about the 40s, we know it's not possible to have a high temperature of 17 with a low temperature of 40.

3. 15 percent—It has to be 15 as we see it will increase to 50; it is impossible to increase from 50 to 15.

4. 50 percent—It has to be 50 as it is impossible to increase from 50 to 15.

5. 13 degrees—While 13 and 30 look the same on the lips, a record low needs to be 13 rather than 30 degrees, especially when the lows the day before were in the 40s.

II. Phoneme and Specific Word Identification

In addition to being able to utilize visual memory and intuitive and synthetic skills, the speechreader needs to be able to quickly recognize speech positions and movements. The following exercises are suggested for practice in recognizing these speech positions or formations as they appear in spoken language.

Exercises:
1. **Consonant Identification—/R/** by Pam Fuller

2. **Rhyming** by Barbara Verspoor

3. **From a Miss to a Mrs.** by Linda Cox Kuntze

4. **Numbers and Initials** by Charles Washko

5. **Slogans** by Alice Bianco

6. **Rooms in a House** by Marlon Kuntze

7. **Which Word Doesn't Belong?** by Elin Dannis

8. **Guess the Sport** by Teresa Hession

Exercise 1. Consonant Identification—/R/

Purpose: To provide practice in recognizing words with an initial /R/.

Materials: vocabulary list
sentences

Procedure: Write the vocabulary on the board and practice it.
Students are to speechread each sentence as the instructor says it, write the sentence, and then underline the vocabulary word.

Vocabulary: receive, remind, relax, realize, recover, recommend, recognize, retest

Sentences:
1. Have you received a letter from your mother?

2. Let's relax awhile.

3. Tom's advisor recommended that he take organic chemistry for his major.

4. Please remind me to go to the class meeting tonight.

5. When Bill didn't pass his driver's test, he had to be retested.

6. The teacher did not recognize her former student.

7. John has recovered from his surgery and has gone back to work.

8. I realize that many students are excited about going home for vacation.

Answers: 1. received; 2. relax; 3. recommended; 4. remind; 5. retested;
6. recognize; 7. recovered; 8. realize

Exercise 2. Rhyming

Purpose: To provide practice in identifying rhyming words.

Materials: paper/pen
sentences

Procedure: The teacher reads the sentences one at a time. The students are instructed to write a word that rhymes with the last word in each sentence. The teacher can say the word or encourage students to think of the answers themselves.

Sentences:
1. An angry employer is a cross _____.
2. An oven is where cookies and cakes _____.
3. On a clear summer night you can see a June _____.
4. A healthy dog is a sound _____.
5. A dark room needs a bright _____.
6. My uncles are my mother's _____.
7. A marathon usually isn't a fun _____.
8. An overfed kitten will become a fat _____.
9. A good play in a card game is a quick _____.
10. Every coach hopes he will have a dream _____.
11. A hen covered with oil is a slick _____.
12. The house with so many animals in it was called Sue's _____.
13. This month's salary is known as May _____.
14. A starving young horse is a bony _____.
15. A recurring injury always seems to gain _____.

Answers: 1. boss; 2. bake; 3. moon; 4. hound; 5. light; 6. brothers; 7. run; 8. cat; 9. trick; 10. team; 11. chick; 12. zoo; 13. pay; 14. pony; 15. pain

Exercise 3. From a Miss to a Mrs.

Purpose: To give practice in rhyming.

Materials: poem

Procedure: Students are instructed to speechread the instructor and fill in the blanks as the appropriate words are said.
Upon completion the instructor will provide the correct rhyming words.

Poem: Miniskirts and hip _____;
Bikini suits and dark _____.

Records, skates, and bongo _____;
Old love letters that she _____.

Riding a cycle, hair in the _____;
Sweat shirts, blue jeans, an occasional _____.

Trying a new hairdo and painting _____;
Impressing her guy, oh, how he _____.

Made up eyes with lashes _____; (a little help this time)
Dancing the jerk and swim, not the _____.

Cheering, gossiping, sharing the _____;
Usually all about the _____.

Sports car, guitars, combos, _____;
Surfing, swimming, lying in the _____.

Parties, dates, skipping a _____;
All these things to a girl _____.

These make the modern girl so _____;
But not her old-fashioned mom and _____!

Husband, sewing, cooking, _____;
All these things turn the _____

MISS INTO A _____.

Answers:

clothes	lips	fun	love
hose	flips	sun	above
boards	false	meal	Mrs.
hoards	waltz	appeal	
breeze	joys	glad	
squeeze	boys	dad	

Exercise 4. Numbers and Initials

Purpose: To provide practice in speechreading numbers and to challenge the student's knowledge and intellect.

Materials: exercise sheet
paper/pen

Procedure: The teacher explains that the students are to write the words that match the initials on the exercise sheet. The numbers should help to identify the words. The teacher will say each set of numbers and words, one at a time. The teacher may provide the answers, or students may share their answers with each other.

Exercise:

4 = q in a g

_____

4 = s of the y

_____

9 = p in the s s

_____

11 = p on a f t

_____

13 = s on the A f

_____

16 = o in a p

_____

18 = h on a g c

_____

26 = l of the a

_____

29 = d in F in a l y

_____

50 = s in A

_____

52 = w in a y

_____

54 = c in a d (with the j)

_____

60 = s in a m

_____

88 = p k

_____

90 = d in a r a

_____

Answers:

quarts in a gallon

seasons of the year

planets in a solar system

players on a football team

stripes on the American flag

ounces in a pound

holes on a golf course

letters of the alphabet

days in February in a leap year

states in America

weeks in a year

cards in a deck (with the jokers)

seconds in a minute

piano keys

degrees in a right angle

Exercise 5. Slogans

Purpose: To provide practice recognizing specific words and phrases.

Materials: answer sheet
            list of slogans

Procedure: Each advertising slogan is spoken by the instructor. The student is to speechread the slogan and then underline the appropriate product on the answer sheet.

Slogans: 1. The uncola

2. Fly the friendly skies of _____.

3. You've come a long way, baby.

4. It is a natural for fresh breath.

5. Everything you always wanted in a beer and less.

6. You deserve a break today.

7. If you aren't getting more, you're getting less.

8. _____ tastes good like a cigarette should.

9. When you are having more than one!

10. I'd rather fight than switch.

11. Come to where the flavor is, come to _____ country.

12. There's a little _____ in every woman.

13. It's the real thing.

Answer Sheet:

1.	7-Up	Cola	Sprite
2.	TWA	Eastern	United
3.	Max	Virginia Slims	Now
4.	Juicy Fruit	Doublemint	Certs
5.	Lite	Miller	Colt 45
6.	Gino's	Hot Shoppes	McDonald's
7.	More	Thin	True
8.	Newport	Kool	Winston
9.	Schaefer	Schlitz	Michelob
10.	Tareyton	Camel	Salem
11.	Kent	Marlboro	Doral
12.	Flower	Lucky Strike	Eve
13.	Pepsi	Tab	Coke

Answers: 1. 7-Up; 2. United; 3. Virginia Slims; 4. Doublemint; 5. Lite; 6. McDonald's; 7. More; 8. Winston; 9. Schaefer; 10. Tareyton; 11. Marlboro; 12. Eve; 13. Coke

Exercise 6. Rooms in a House

Purpose: To practice identifying specific words.

Materials: paper/pen
list of clue words

Procedure: Students are to speechread each set of clue words to determine which room is being identified and then write the name of the room on their paper.

Clue Words:
1. bed, dresser, nightstand, pillow, mattress
2. stove, oven, refrigerator, sink, dishwasher
3. sofa, coffee table, lamps, television set, fireplace
4. shower, bathtub, toilet, sink
5. junk, trunks, storage
6. workshop, furnace, water heater, storage
7. table, candles, tablecloth, silverware, chairs
8. car, workbench, tools, lawnmower
9. Ping-Pong table, chess table, pool table, games
10. clothes, hangers, towels, linens
11. dishes, utensils, pots and pans, canned food
12. rooms, doors, windows, roof, floors

Answers: 1. bedroom; 2. kitchen; 3. living room; 4. bathroom; 5. attic; 6. basement; 7. dining room; 8. garage; 9. game room; 10. closet; 11. pantry; 12. house

Exercise 7. Which Word Doesn't Belong?

Purpose: To provide mind training while requiring word recognition.

Materials: word groups
paper/pen

Procedure: Students speechread all the words in a group, find the one word that doesn't fit, and write that word on their paper.

Word Groups:
1. chalk, erase, pencil, pen, paintbrush
2. duck, pig, dog, chicken, turkey
3. milk, bread, water, gasoline, rubbing alcohol
4. bottle, wastebasket, rock, bucket, gas tank

5. hen, rooster, girl, mother, queen

6. London, Paris, Rome, New York, Washington

7. tree, whale, fish, grass, coal

8. total, pile, sum, penny, group

9. airplane, racing car, space capsule, bird, bat

10. lamb, flock, shepherd, cow, cowboy

11. sheep, cow, pig, pork, calf

12. horse, cow, deer, goat, mule

13. cot, chair, couch, bed, hammock

14. Brazil, France, Germany, Poland, Denmark

15. train, car, tractor, airplane, harvester

16. sheep, fawn, colt, calf, cub

17. wolf, buffalo, pig, coyote, deer

18. funeral, wedding, graduation, party, picnic

Answers:

1. erase	6. New York	11. pork	16. sheep
2. dog	7. coal	12. deer	17. pig
3. bread	8. penny	13. chair	18. funeral
4. rock	9. racing car	14. Brazil	
5. rooster	10. flock	15. airplane	

Exercise 8. Guess the Sport

Purpose:	To practice speechreading specific words in order to identify a sport.
Materials:	list of words
	paper/pen
Procedure:	The students speechread the clue words and tell or write the appropriate sport.
Clue Words:	1. Colts, rough, beer, touchdown, shoulderpads
	2. wet, refreshing, standing on water, ski
	3. ball, racquet, court, love
	4. hoop, court, dribble, gym
	5. laps, freestyle, backstroke, chlorine

6. split, tumble, horse, balance beam

7. pole, bait, boat, hook

8. hot dog, crowd, Yankees, home run

Answers: 1. football; 2. waterskiing; 3. tennis; 4. basketball; 5. swimming; 6. gymnastics; 7. fishing; 8. baseball

III. Games and Quizzes

The following exercises were developed to provide practice in speechreading connected material to obtain specific information. In order to be successful at these exercises, the student must recognize clue words and phrases and use context to answer specific questions. Intuitive synthetic skill development, rather than literal word recognition, is stressed. The topics used in the games and quizzes are of interest to most adults and adolescents.

Exercises:
1. **Everyday Situations** by Mary Johnstone
2. **Seasons** by Ellie Korres and Richard Baldi
3. **What's the Word?** by Ruth Dunham Walker
4. **Our Presidents** by Bob Firestone, Rene Poyer Suiter, and Ken Roth
5. **U.S. History and Geography** by Jim Perry
6. **More U.S. History and Geography** by Steven Blehm
7. **What Young Adults Enjoy Doing** by Tammy Timmons Opperman
8. **Find the Animal** by Joel Marcus
9. **Professions** by Danny Noling
10. **Name the Birds** by Eugene Eabon
11. **Occupations** by Cherie Sussman
12. **Name the /R/ Word** by Linda McNeil

Exercise 1. Everyday Situations

Purpose: To have the student practice speechreading questions that are usually asked in commonly experienced situations.

Materials: slips of paper, each identifying a situation and providing a clue statement list of questions for each situation

Procedure: Each student draws a slip of paper containing a situation and clue. The instructor asks the student to identify the situation and then asks the appropriate questions. The student speechreads the questions and answers them.

Situations: **Dentist's Office** (receptionist)

Clue statement: It is a first visit.

1. Have you had an appointment with the doctor before?

2. Will you please fill out this card?

3. Do you have dental insurance?

4. Do you want to have your teeth cleaned?

5. Will you pay now, or shall I send you a bill?

6. How soon would you like another appointment?

Shoe Store
Clue statement: The clerk approaches you.

1. Hello, what kind of shoes do you have in mind?

2. What size do you wear?

3. How do they feel—comfortable or too tight?

4. We don't have these in brown. Would you like to see them in tan?

5. Do you prefer a lower heel?

6. Will that be cash or charge?

Beauty Salon
Clue statement: You have asked for a cut and styling.

1. Is there anyone special you want to cut your hair?

2. Do you want a razor cut or scissors cut?

3. Do you like your bangs cut straight across or uneven?

4. Do you want me to taper it in the back or a blunt cut?

5. Can you bend your head down, please?

6. Do you want me to blow dry your hair when I'm finished?

Airport
Clue statement: You want to make reservations to fly home.

1. Do you want an early flight or later in the day?

2. Do you prefer to sit next to the window or on the aisle?

3. Do you want smoking or nonsmoking?

4. Will you need transportation from the airport to town?

5. Can you be at the airport one hour before flight time?

6. Are you going to buy your ticket now or pick it up later?

Restaurant
Clue statement: You must communicate with the host/hostess and waiter/waitress.

1. How many are in your group?

2. Do you want a table near the window?

3. Will you have something to drink before dinner?

4. Are you going to check your coat?

5. What kind of dressing do you want on your salad?

6. Baked potato, mashed, or french fries?

Exercise 2. Seasons

Purpose: To provide practice using clue words to aid in topic identification.

Materials: sentences about the four seasons
paper/pen (if desired)

Procedure: The students will look for clue words while the instructor reads the sentences to help them identify which season is being described.

Students may be asked to name the season or to state which word(s) helped them choose the season or both.

Sentences:
1. Daffodils are my favorite flowers.

2. I love to watch ice-skating.

3. She will be 17 years old in October.

4. I have a painful sunburn on my back.

5. Our football team won.

6. I'm glad school is almost over.

7. My grandfather looked like Santa Claus.

8. We often go to the beach.

9. We had a picnic Easter Sunday.

10. It's difficult to drive on icy roads.

11. My birthday is November 1st.

12. Are you going swimming in the lake tomorrow?

13. I like to watch the fireworks on July 4th.

14. The grass has finally become green now.

15. We stayed up late New Year's Eve.

16. The leaves started to fall off the trees.

17. I received many presents for Christmas.

18. Her bikini cost twenty dollars.

19. He dressed as a ghost for Halloween.

20. Did you notice her new fur coat?

Answers/Clue Words:

1. spring/daffodils
2. winter/ice-skating
3. autumn/October
4. summer/sunburn
5. autumn/football
6. spring/school-over
7. winter/Santa Claus
8. summer/beach
9. spring/Easter Sunday
10. winter/icy roads
11. autumn/November
12. summer/swimming, lake
13. summer/July 4th, fireworks
14. spring/grass, green
15. winter/New Year's Eve
16. autumn/leaves started to fall
17. winter/presents, Christmas
18. summer/bikini
19. autumn/Halloween, ghost
20. winter/fur coat

Sentences and Phrases:

1. Birds are singing in the air.

2. A scarecrow is in the cornfield.

3. A countryside covered with white powder

4. Swimming at your favorite beach

5. Leaves of different colors

6. Flowers blooming, happy bees

7. Let's go ice-skating on the lake.

8. We need to turn on the air conditioner.

9. A time to get a suntan

10. If you go camping, watch for bears.

11. Time for school again

12. A time when it's hard to concentrate or study

13. A time for sweaters

14. Have a Merry Christmas and a Happy New Year.

15. College students can't wait for this season at the end of the school year.

Answers/Clue Words:

1. spring/birds singing
2. autumn/scarecrow, cornfield
3. winter/covered with white powder
4. summer/swimming, beach
5. autumn/leaves, different colors
6. spring/flowers blooming
7. winter/ice-skating
8. summer/air conditioner
9. summer/suntan
10. summer/camping, bears
11. autumn/school again
12. spring/hard to concentrate or study
13. autumn/sweaters
14. winter/Christmas, New Year
15. spring/end of school year

Exercise 3. What's the Word?

Purpose: To provide practice in understanding unrelated sentences or phrases.

Materials: answer sheets
descriptions to be identified

Procedure: Instruct the students to write answers to the descriptions on the answer sheets. If a student understands the description but does not know the answer, the instructor may give the answer for speechreading practice.

Descriptions:
1. The opposite of up

2. The material of elephant tusks

3. Usually eaten for breakfast

4. When on the beach, you need to watch for high _____.

5. Don't forget to _____ me in your plans.

6. Work hard, but don't _____ it.

7. Close at hand; live close

8. The United States has both a navy and an _____.

9. Some people like _____ bread.

10. However; still

Answer Sheet:

(See if you can find six words reading down)

D
I
C
T
I
O
N
A
R
Y

Descriptions:
1. A headgear with no bit

2. When a horse is feeling frisky, we say the horse is "feeling its _____."

3. Two leather straps used to guide the horse

4. Put on the horse's back for people to sit in

5. The same as number four but is very flat

6. We put our foot in this

7. Put on the horse's body to help it pull heavy equipment

8. Putting the horse out to pasture when it becomes _____

9. Lots of people love horses, _____ me.

10. What is a father horse called?

Answer Sheet: H

(Reading down, O
can you find an insect R
that is noted for
its hard work?) S

E

S

H

O

E

S

Answers:

1. down   1. halter
2. ivory   2. oats
3. cereal   3. reins
4. tide   4. saddle
5. include   5. English
6. overdo   6. stirrup
7. nearby   7. harness
8. army   8. old
9. rye   9. especially
10. yet   10. sire

vein, very, word, reel, do, met   ant

Exercise 4. Our Presidents

Purpose: To provide practice in speechreading connected speech.

Materials: questions containing well-known and not so well-known facts about U.S. presidents

Procedure: This may be conducted as a game with teams, or students may be asked to write the answers if they know them. If a student understands the question but doesn't know the answer, he or she may be asked to write the question. Flexibility is the key.

Questions:
1. Who was the youngest president to be elected?
2. Who was the first president whose mother was alive when he was inaugurated?
3. Who was the first president to reside in Washington, D.C.?
4. Who was the first president to be born in a log cabin?
5. Who was the first widower to be inaugurated as president?
6. Who was the first Boy Scout to become president?
7. Who was the tallest president?
8. Who was the first Democratic president elected after the Civil War?
9. Which president served in office for only one month?
10. Who was the first president to take the oath of office in an airplane?
11. Who was the last president whose term of office expired on March 3?
12. Who was the first president to become chief justice of the U.S.?
13. Who was the only president to serve as Speaker of the House?
14. Who was the largest president?
15. Which president held the first presidential press conference?
16. Who was the only president to be married in the White House?
17. Which presidents are buried in Arlington National Cemetery?
18. Who was the only president who was a bachelor?
19. What two former presidents died on the same day?
20. Which president lived the longest?
21. Which president had the most children?
22. Who was the first president to speak on the radio?
23. Who was the first president to appear on television?
24. Who was the last president to ride to his inauguration in a horse-drawn carriage?
25. Which president died the youngest?
26. Who was the president when the Great Depression began?
27. Which president was the first Roman Catholic to hold office as president?
28. Who served the longest time as president?
29. From which state have the most presidents come?

Answers:

1. Teddy Roosevelt
2. George Washington
3. John Adams
4. Andrew Jackson (in S.C.)
5. Thomas Jefferson
6. John F. Kennedy (JFK)
7. Abraham Lincoln
8. Grover Cleveland
9. William Harrison
10. Lyndon B. Johnson (LBJ)
11. Herbert Hoover
12. William H. Taft

13. James Polk
14. Taft (weighed more than 300 pounds and stood 6 feet 2 inches tall)
15. Woodrow Wilson (March 15, 1913)
16. Grover Cleveland
17. Taft and JFK
18. James Buchanan
19. John Adams and Thomas Jefferson
20. Harry S. Truman

21. John Tyler
22. Woodrow Wilson
23. Franklin D. Roosevelt (FDR)
24. Woodrow Wilson
25. JFK
26. Herbert Hoover
27. JFK
28. FDR
29. Virginia

Exercise 5. U.S. History and Geography

Purpose: To practice speechreading connected materials to obtain enough information to answer multiple-choice questions.

Materials: questions
answer sheets

Procedure: Students speechread questions about U.S. history and geography and circle the correct answer on the answer sheet. If a student does not know the answer but understands the question, he or she may repeat or write the question.

Questions:
1. Who was the 15th president of the U.S.?
2. In which state is Santa Fe?
3. Olympia is the capital of _____.
4. The largest state in the U.S. is _____.
5. The Mason-Dixon line is located between which two states?
6. _____ was the president of the U.S. during the "Era of Good Feeling."
7. _____ killed Alexander Hamilton in a duel.
8. The capital of Minnesota is _____.
9. Which president wrote the well-known document known as the Roosevelt Corollary?
10. _____ was her maiden name before she married Franklin Roosevelt.

Answer Sheet:
1. (a) Andrew Johnson
   (b) Abraham Lincoln
   (c) James Buchanan

2. (a) New Mexico
   (b) New Jersey
   (c) New Hampshire

3. (a) Oregon
   (b) Washington
   (c) Idaho

4. (a) Alaska
   (b) Texas
   (c) California

5. (a) North Carolina/South Carolina
   (b) Maryland/Pennsylvania
   (c) Virginia/Maryland

6. (a) Andrew Jackson
   (b) James Madison
   (c) James Monroe

7. (a) Aaron Burr
   (b) Henry Clay
   (c) John Adams

8. (a) Minneapolis
   (b) St. Paul
   (c) Bloomington

9. (a) Teddy Roosevelt
   (b) Franklin Roosevelt
   (c) James Monroe

10. (a) Eleanor Delano
    (b) Eleanor Garretson
    (c) Eleanor Roosevelt

Answers: 1. c; 2. a; 3. b; 4. a; 5. b; 6. c; 7. a; 8. b.; 9. a; 10. c

Exercise 6. More U.S. History and Geography

Purpose: To provide more practice in speechreading facts and statements about U.S. history and geography.

Materials: paper/pencils
questions

Procedure: Students number their papers from 1–10. The teacher then reads the questions one at a time, and the students write the answers. Upon completion of the exercise, the teacher tells the students to write the last letter of the first word in each answer on their papers. If their answers are correct, they will have spelled *lipreading*.

Questions:
1. Who made the midnight ride to warn about the coming of the British to Boston? (first and last names)
2. What is the longest river in the U.S.?
3. How did the settlers come to America from their countries in the sixteenth century?
4. What is the name of the ship that arrived in Plymouth in 1620?
5. Who was the first president of the U.S.? (first and last names)
6. Name the state that eight U.S. presidents have come from.
7. Who was the first president to resign? (first and last names)
8. Which was the 50th state to join the U.S.?
9. Which country sent men to South America and Mexico to find gold?
10. From where did Benjamin Franklin get electricity with his kite and key?

Answers:

1. Pau*l* Revere
2. Mississipp*i* River
3. shi*p*
4. Mayflowe*r*
5. Georg*e* Washington
6. Virgini*a*
7. Richar*d* Nixon
8. Hawai*i*
9. Spai*n*
10. lightni*ng*

124

Exercise 7. What Young Adults Enjoy Doing

Purpose: To provide practice in understanding and identifying activities and activity-related terminology.

Materials: paper/pen
descriptions of activity to be identified

Procedure: The instructor reads the descriptions and instructs the students to write down the activity or activity-related words. Upon completion, students are told to look for the hidden message to be found by looking at the first letter of each answer. (*Have a nice summer.*)

Descriptions:
1. Taking a long walk or walking through rural areas for pleasure
2. Having to do with movement or actions
3. A game in which players hit a ball with their hands so that it goes back and forth across a high net
4. Traveling for the purpose of discovery
5. An exciting or remarkable experience
6. A place for dancing, eating, and entertainment; open only at night
7. A house or building designed for inside sports
8. People living in tents near a lake or in the woods during the summer
9. Activities used to give training and to cause figure improvement
10. Moving through water by moving arms and legs
11. Where scuba divers and snorkelers look for shells
12. A building where works of art or other objects are kept and displayed
13. The showing of a motion picture
14. Something young people are always looking for
15. Used to hit a ball for tennis and badminton

Answers:

1. *h*iking
2. *a*ctivities
3. *v*olleyball
4. *e*xploring
5. *a*dventure
6. *n*ight club
7. *i*ndoor arena
8. *c*amping
9. *e*xercises
10. *s*wimming
11. *u*nder water
12. *m*useum
13. *m*ovies
14. *e*xcitement
15. *r*acquet

Have a nice summer.

Exercise 8. Find the Animal

Purpose: To provide practice in using synthetic and intuitive skills as well as clue words.

Materials: paper/pen
sentences

Procedure: Students are informed that each sentence to be read is about an animal. They are to write down the name of the animal in each sentence. Upon completion, the students are told to read the first letter of each animal and find the hidden word. (*lipreading*)

Sentences:

1. The roar of the *lion* is very loud.

2. In Africa the *impala* runs very fast over the grass.

3. We have two very cute *pandas* from China at the zoo now.

4. Did you know that *raccoons* always wash their food before they eat it?

5. The symbol of the United States is the *eagle*.

6. *Apes* are very intelligent.

7. People shoot *deer* for food.

8. There are many kinds of *insects* flying in the air.

9. Can you hear the song of a *nightingale*?

10. A *giraffe* has the longest neck of all animals.

Answers:

1.	*l*ion	7.	*d*eer
2.	*i*mpala	8.	*i*nsects
3.	*p*andas	9.	*n*ightingale
4.	*r*accoons	10.	*g*iraffe
5.	*e*agle		*lipreading*
6.	*a*pes		

Exercise 9. Professions

Purpose: To identify professions by understanding clue words in descriptive phrases.

Materials: descriptive phrases
paper/pen

Procedure: The students name the profession of each descriptive phrase as it is read. The answers may be written or given verbally if teams are used.

Descriptive Phrases: 1. person who designs buildings

2. man who arrests criminals

3. person who drives passengers from city to city or state to state

4. person who argues during court sessions

5. builder who uses a hammer, nails, and saw

6. person who treats or operates on patients in a hospital

7. person who flies airplanes

8. person who works in a mine

9. person who gives grades for tests

10. woman who cleans house

11. person who fixes cars

12. person who bawls out the players during games

13. men who put out fires

14. person who performs stunts

15. person who works with electric wires

16. person who makes brick walls

17. person who makes kids of all ages laugh

18. person who sneaks into another country to discover secrets

19. men who rode spaceships to the moon

20. person who takes shorthand and types letters

Answers:

1.	architect	11.	auto mechanic
2.	policeman	12.	coach
3.	bus driver	13.	firemen
4.	lawyer	14.	daredevil
5.	carpenter	15.	electrician
6.	doctor	16.	bricklayer
7.	pilot	17.	clown
8.	miner	18.	spy
9.	teacher	19.	astronauts
10.	housewife	20.	secretary

Exercise 10. Name the Birds

Purpose: To provide practice in speechreading sentences to gain information.

Materials: paper/pen
sentences describing birds

Procedure: The teacher reads the descriptions, and the students write the name of each bird being described. This can be conducted as competition between teams or as an individual exercise.

Sentences:
1. One of the first signs of springtime; has a red breast and likes to eat worms
2. A familiar domestic bird found on the farm
3. A symbol of peace and the Holy Spirit in the Christian religion
4. Represents the United States government and American freedom
5. A tiny bird that flies like a bee
6. A water bird with a short neck that is usually served with an orange glaze in restaurants
7. A bird with the same name as a churchman in the Vatican; likes to eat sunflower seeds
8. The largest bird in the world; cannot fly and lives in Africa
9. A short, fat bird; lives in the subfreezing temperatures of the South Pole and has the same name as Batman's foe
10. A bird usually served with stuffing and hot gravy and eaten after thanks is given
11. The emblem of the National Broadcasting Company
12. A bird found in the Amazon jungle and the legendary pet of pirates

Answers:

1. robin
2. chicken
3. dove
4. eagle
5. hummingbird
6. duck

7. cardinal
8. ostrich
9. penguin
10. turkey
11. peacock
12. parrot

Exercise 11. Occupations

Purpose: To practice utilizing intuitive skills.

Materials: answer sheet
descriptions of occupations

Procedure: Students are to match the descriptions read by the teacher with the occupations on their answer sheets by writing the number of the description in the blank by the occupation.

Descriptions: 1. You must make an appointment with me.
I help to keep your body in good health.

2. I work on the stage.
I play the part of other people.

3. I live in the dorm.
I enforce student life rules.

4. I'm a very lonely man.
I rarely get a chance to fix our washers and dryers.

5. I defend criminals.
I may also work on divorces.

6. I may have a Ph.D.
I help people with their mental well-being.

7. I take pictures.
I may be a free-lance artist.

8. I lie well.
I usually get elected to office.

9. I use a lot of water in my job.
I see a lot of leftover food.

10. I work with languages.
I may do quite a bit of research.

Answer Sheet: ____ doctor

____ lawyer

____ teacher

____ interpreter

____ residence advisor

____ butcher

____ foreman

____ dentist

____ secretary

____ social worker

____ psychologist

____ Maytag repairman

____ chemist

____ computer programmer

____ film producer

____ actor/actress

____ waitress/waiter

____ photographer

____ salesperson

____ politician

____ linguist

____ dishwasher

Answers:

1. doctor
2. actor/actress
3. residence advisor
4. Maytag repairman
5. lawyer

6. psychologist
7. photographer
8. politician
9. dishwasher
10. linguist

Exercise 12. Name the /R/ Word

Purpose: To provide practice in speechreading sentences that require responses involving initial /R/.

Materials: sentences (or commands) describing activities or items that begin with /R/ chalkboard or flip chart to record points

Procedure: Form two teams. Instruct the teams that they must speechread each sentence and respond with words which begin with /R/. An incorrect response will result in no points and loss of a turn.

Sentences:
1. Name something that is vacuumed weekly by good housekeepers.

2. Name something that a cook or baker uses to make pie crusts.

3. Name something that little girls love to use for jumping up and down.

4. Name something that we do with a newspaper or a book.

5. Name something that people do when they are tired.

6. Name something that is used to keep food cold.

7. Name a person who steals money.

8. Name an animal that loves to eat carrots.

9. Name something that people do when they quit working or become older.

10. Name a sport that requires a court, a small racquet, and a ball.

Answers:

1. rug	6. refrigerator
2. rolling pin	7. robber
3. rope	8. rabbit
4. read	9. retire
5. rest	10. racquet ball

IV. Paragraphs and Related Sentences

Understanding continuous discourse requires that the speechreader make use of visual memory skills as well as situational cues to predict or anticipate what might come next. The following exercises are designed to train these skills.

Exercises:

1. **Stories and Questions:** *My Pet Dog* and *A Bus Trip* by Mary Johnstone; *Swimming Lessons* and *A Day at the Museum* by Heather Bouten

2. **A New York Trip** by Rosie Yuch

3. **How to Bathe a Dog** by Elin Dannis

4. **Canada** by Macklin Youngs

5. **Who and What Am I?** by Elin Dannis

6. **What's the Holiday?** by Mary Jessen

7. **Animals—What Am I?** by Robbie Carmichael

Exercise 1. Stories and Questions

Purpose: To identify the topic and to answer questions about short paragraphs that are read by the teacher.

Materials: four short stories with questions

Procedure: The teacher reads one story at a time to the students. Students identify the topic of each story and explain what clues they used. Then the questions are read, one at a time, with students responding when they think they have the right answer. If a question is answered incorrectly, other students are given a turn until someone answers correctly.

Story One: **My Pet Dog**

When I was a little girl, I had a pet dog. The dog was very smart, and I taught him to do many tricks. He could sit up, roll over, and bring in the newspaper. When anyone knocked on the door, the dog would bark and wag his tail. If he wanted to go outside for a walk, he would stand on his back legs and put his paws on the doorknob.

Questions: What was the topic of the story? How do you know?

1. When did I have this pet dog?

2. What tricks could he do?

3. When did he bark and wag his tail?

4. How did I know if he wanted to go for a walk?

Answers:

1. when I was a little girl
2. sit up, roll over, bring in the newspaper
3. when anyone knocked on the door
4. if he stood on his back legs and put his paws on the doorknob

Story Two: **A Bus Trip**

Last summer we took a trip by bus. We traveled all through the western part of the United States. We saw many interesting cities and stopped in Denver, Las Vegas, and San Francisco. The bus was air-conditioned so it was never uncomfortable. When it was time to eat, we usually stopped at a fast-food restaurant along the highway.

Questions: What was the topic of the story? How do you know this?

1. What area of the United States did we travel through?
2. What three interesting cities did we stop in?
3. Why was the bus never uncomfortable?
4. What did we usually do when it was time to eat?

Answers:

1. the western part
2. Denver, Las Vegas, San Francisco
3. it was air-conditioned
4. stopped at a fast-food restaurant along the highway

Story Three: **Swimming Lessons**

A group of boys and girls are taking swimming lessons now. They are learning the front crawl, back crawl, breast stroke, and side stroke. They go for two hours every morning except Saturdays and Sundays for three weeks. On the last day, they will each be given an examination, and if they pass, they will receive a certificate.

Questions: What is the topic of the story? How do you know?

1. What are the boys and girls taking now?
2. What are they learning?
3. How often do they go?
4. How long do the lessons last?
5. What will they get if they pass the examination?

Answers:

1. swimming lessons
2. front crawl, back crawl, breast stroke, side stroke
3. every morning except Saturdays and Sundays for three weeks
4. two hours
5. a certificate

Story Four: **A Day at the Museum**

We went to the museum last Saturday. We saw prehistoric animals, primitive cultures, and the history of transportation. We spent the whole day there. At the end of the day we were exhausted and had sore feet. We decided to go home and take a hot bath.

Questions: What was the topic of the story? How do you know?

1. Where did we go?
2. What did we see?
3. How long were we at the museum?
4. How did we feel at the end of the day?
5. What did we do when we arrived home?

Answers:

1. the museum
2. prehistoric animals, primitive cultures, history of transportation
3. all day
4. exhausted, sore feet
5. took a hot bath

Exercise 2. A New York Trip

Purpose: To provide experience in speechreading continuous narration and to improve visual memory.

Materials: story
multiple-choice questions

Procedure: The instructor reads the story. The students answer questions upon completion of the story. If necessary, the instructor may repeat the story.

Story: Yesterday David went to New York with his parents. They were in the city all day. In the morning they went to a museum. David saw some beautiful paintings. His mother liked the pictures of women and children. David liked an interesting picture of an old man.

At one o'clock David was hungry. He and his parents ate lunch in a restaurant. The waiter was friendly, and the food was excellent. David ordered soup, chicken, and potatoes. His mother and father ordered fish. They drank coffee, but David drank milk.

After lunch David's mother went to the library. David and his father went to the circus. The clowns were funny. They saw short and tall clowns. Some clowns were old and some were young. One old clown had big hands and feet. David liked the circus.

At seven o'clock David and his parents went to a small, quiet restaurant. They ate dinner with some friends. David was hungry and tired. It was a busy day.

Questions: 1. When did David go to New York?   a. last week
                                                        b. yesterday
                                                        c. at one o'clock

              2. What did David see in the museum?   a. an old man
                                                        b. some paintings
                                                        c. a friendly waiter

              3. Where did David and his parents eat lunch?   a. at the museum
                                                              b. with friends
                                                              c. in a restaurant

              4. When did they eat lunch?   a. in the morning
                                                        b. before 12 o'clock
                                                        c. at one o'clock

              5. What kind of a man was the waiter?   a. old
                                                        b. friendly
                                                        c. hungry

              6. What did David eat?   a. fish
                                                        b. chicken
                                                        c. an egg

              7. How was the food?   a. excellent
                                                        b. cold
                                                        c. beautiful

              8. What did David's mother drink?   a. coffee
                                                        b. cold milk
                                                        c. water

              9. Where did David's mother go in the afternoon?   a. to the circus
                                                                 b. to the library
                                                                 c. home

             10. When did David and his father go to the circus?   a. after lunch
                                                                    b. at seven o'clock
                                                                    c. after dinner

             11. What did they see at the circus?   a. some friends
                                                        b. David's mother
                                                        c. clowns

             12. What kind of clowns were they?   a. tired
                                                        b. busy
                                                        c. funny

13. Where did David go after the circus?

a. to the library
b. to a restaurant
c. home

14. What kind of restaurant was it?

a. small
b. busy
c. big

15. Who went to the restaurant?

a. David went alone
b. David and his father
c. David, his parents, and friends

Answers:

1. b	6. b	11. c
2. b	7. a	12. c
3. c	8. a	13. b
4. c	9. b	14. a
5. b	10. a	15. c

Exercise 3. How to Bathe a Dog

Purpose: To speechread continuous discourse about a specific topic to be able to answer questions.

Materials: story
questions and answers

Procedure: The instructor reads the story as many times as necessary for all students to understand it. The questions are asked; they may be answered either orally or in writing.

Story: When bathing a dog, you should use only soap made for dogs. This type of soap is better because it gets rid of the dog's fleas. A warm place, such as the basement sink, needs to be found so the dog won't catch a cold. Wet the dog thoroughly and bathe it with the dog soap and a brush. After soaping the dog, rinse it well until all the soap is gone and the dog is clean. Take the dog out of the water, wrap some old towels around it, and rub it well. If you have a hair dryer, use it to dry the dog while brushing it. Brush the dog's coat until it is shiny and dry.

Questions: What is the topic of the story? (optional)

1. What kind of soap should you use when bathing a dog?

2. Why is dog soap better for dogs than regular body soap?

3. What kind of a place should you find to bathe a dog? Why?

4. What is the first thing that should be done?

5. What items are needed to bathe a dog?

6. What should be done after a dog has been bathed?

7. How can a dog be dried?

8. How can you tell whether or not the dog is dry?

Answers:

1. soap made for dogs
2. gets rid of fleas
3. a warm place;
   so it won't catch cold
4. wet the dog thoroughly

5. soap, towel, hair dryer, brush
6. wrap it in a towel and rub well
7. with a towel and a hair dryer
8. when its coat is clean and shiny

Exercise 4. Canada

Purpose: To provide training of visual memory and ability to understand connected material.

Materials: paper/pen
paragraph
questions

Procedure: After explaining, using full voice and/or sign language, that the paragraph is about Canada, the teacher reads it to the students. The students are to answer questions about Canada based on the material read by the teacher.

Paragraph: Canada is the second largest country in the world, including its fresh water area. It is made up of ten provinces. The capital city is Ottawa. Canada is more than 100 years old. Its confederacy was founded in 1869. The first prime minister was John A. McDonald. A long-time, popular prime minister was Pierre Trudeau. Canada is renowned for its nickel, lumber, and uranium deposits. It has the longest highway in the world, the Trans-Canada Highway, that stretches from Vancouver, B.C., to Newfoundland. From time to time there are problems in governance. One of these problems is with the separatist movement in Quebec. In Canada the only kind of air or water pollution you can see is marked "manufactured in the United States." Canada is a beautiful place to live and work. It is free of the problems that ravage the rest of the world. It is free of the racial riots of the United States and other countries.

Questions: 1. What is the second largest country in the world?

2. How many provinces does Canada have?

3. What is the capital of Canada?

4. How old is Canada?

5. When was the confederacy of Canada founded?

6. Who was the first prime minister?

7. Who was a long-time, popular prime minister?

8. What are the resources for which Canada is renowned?

9. From what two points does the Trans-Canada Highway start and end?

10. In what province does the separatist movement occur?

Answers:

1. Canada
2. ten
3. Ottawa
4. more than 100 years
5. 1869

6. John A. McDonald
7. Pierre Trudeau
8. nickel, lumber, uranium
9. Vancouver, B.C., Newfoundland
10. Quebec

Exercise 5. Who and What Am I?

Purpose: To provide practice in understanding continuous dialogue.

Materials: paper/pen
sentences describing the person or item to be identified

Procedure: Students are instructed to write who or what is described by the instructor.

Descriptions:
1. I am soft.
   You put your head on me.
   I am usually found on a bed.
2. I have a long neck.
   I have no voice.
   I am very tall.
   I like to eat leaves off the trees.
3. I have a face.
   I have two hands.
   I have no eyes.
   I tell you the time.
4. I am very cold.
   I am in the kitchen.
   People put food in me.

5. You carry me when it rains.
   You must open me up.
   I keep you dry.
6. I pump you up in a chair.
   I fix your teeth.
   Sometimes I give you a shot.
7. I am small.
   I can open a door.
   I can start a car.
8. I work in a hospital.
   I wear a white uniform.
   I help the doctor.
9. I am on the floor.
   I am soft.
   People like to walk on me.

10. We hang at windows.
    We are long.
    We are beautiful.
11. I have a small tail.
    I am brown or white.

    I can hop very fast.
    I like to eat carrots.
12. I am in the living room.
    People turn me off and on.
    People like to watch me.

Answers: 1. pillow; 2. giraffe; 3. clock; 4. icebox or refrigerator; 5. umbrella; 6. dentist; 7. key; 8. nurse; 9. rug or carpet; 10. drapes; 11. rabbit; 12. television

Exercise 6. What's the Holiday?

Purpose: To use recognition of clue words to identify the holiday that is discussed.

Materials: list of holidays (may be omitted if not needed by students)
short paragraphs about the following holidays: Christmas, July 4th, Thanksgiving, Halloween, Valentine's Day, Easter, and New Year's

Procedure: If necessary, the holidays are written on the chalkboard and students practice the vocabulary before doing the exercise. Advanced students should identify the holidays without using a list. The students identify the holiday for each paragraph that is read by the instructor.

Paragraphs: On Friday night I went to the shopping mall to visit Santa. I had my picture taken with Santa and one of his elves. On Candy Cane Lane all the stores were decorated with many different kinds of decorations and ornaments.

We celebrated at our picnic with a blast. The sky was full of bright colors. There were Roman candles, sizzles, cherry bombs, and snakes. Our community always has a wonderful display of fireworks during the evening on Independence Day.

The turkey, cranberries, stuffing, pie, and nuts were all so delicious. The family shared their thoughts and prayers of thankfulness.

Every year I look forward to carving a jack-o'-lantern. Trick or treaters always come to the door dressed in the most unusual costumes. Some of them are scary and some are cute. There are always ghosts.

I received a beautiful card with a large red heart in the middle. The card said, "Will you be mine?" This special day is February 14, and there are always many sweetheart balls during this time.

Dyeing eggs different colors and decorating them with flowers, crosses, and other designs is a family fun activity. Hunting for the eggs is a lot of fun for both young and old people.

When the clock strikes twelve at midnight, folks begin to sing Auld Lang Syne and toast each other. They blow noise makers. Many people make resolutions such as quitting smoking or going on a diet.

Answers:

Christmas	Halloween	New Year's
July 4th	Valentine's Day	
Thanksgiving	Easter	

Exercise 7. Animals—What Am I?

Purpose: To provide practice in speechreading continued discourse.

Materials: list of animals
sentences describing animals

Procedure: Write the list of animals on the chalkboard. This may be omitted for more advanced students. The teacher reads each animal description. The students tell which animal is being described. This exercise can be conducted as a game with teams.

Animal List:

beaver	frog	polar bear
bee	kangaroo	shark
deer	monkey	snake
elephant	mouse	squirrel
fox	ostrich	tiger

Animal Descriptions:

1. I live in the North Pole. I am white. I love cold weather.
2. I am small and usually gray. I have a long skinny tail. I love to eat cheese.
3. I hop all day long with my babies in my pouch. Australia is my home.
4. I live in the woods. I have long antlers. I eat fruit, leaves, and tree bark.
5. With my long tail I swing from tree to tree. I live in the jungle, eating free bananas.
6. I am very clever. That is why, when hunted by dog and people, I am hard to catch.
7. I have a bushy tail. I live in a tree. I love to eat nuts.
8. I work hard all the time. I build dams in the water. With my two long front teeth, I collect the necessary wood.
9. I buzz about from flower to flower. My wings are so fast they are hard to see. I never stop working hour after hour. I go here and there collecting nectar for you and me.
10. I have big ears and a long nose. My tusks are made of ivory. Africa is where I roam.

11. I am a good hunter. With my stripes I blend well into my surroundings. I am in the cat family.

12. The ocean is my home. I am strong and swim fast. Many people are afraid of me because of my sharp, pointed teeth. They made me look like a monster in a popular movie.

13. I jump from one lily pod to another. I have big bulging eyes. I have a very fast tongue. With my tongue I snatch and eat a variety of insects.

14. No, I am not slimy, but I do love to crawl and wind my way through the tall grass. I do help people by eating some of their pests. I am long and slender.

15. I cannot fly, but I can run very fast. I protect myself by kicking with my strong legs. I am able to get food with my long neck. Some people think that I love to put my head in the sand.

Answers:

1.	polar bear	6.	fox	11.	tiger
2.	mouse	7.	squirrel	12.	shark
3.	kangaroo	8.	beaver	13.	frog
4.	deer	9.	bee	14.	snake
5.	monkey	10.	elephant	15.	ostrich

References

Alpiner, J. G. (1982). *Handbook of adult rehabilitative audiology* (2nd ed.). Baltimore, MD: Williams & Wilkins.

Alpiner, J. G., Chevrette, W., Glascoe, G., Metz, M., & Olsen, B. (1982). The Denver scale of communication function. In J. G. Alpiner (Ed.), *Handbook of adult rehabilitative audiology* (2nd ed., pp. 46–49). Baltimore, MD: Williams & Wilkins.

Bally, S. J., Wilson, M. P., & Bergan, J. (1984). *Effective communication strategies: A guide for the hearing-impaired.* Unpublished manuscript.

Berger, K. W. (1972). Visemes and homophenous words. *Teacher of the Deaf, 70,* 369–399.

Berger, K. W. (1978). *Speechreading, principles and methods* (2nd ed.). Kent, OH: National Educational Press, Inc.

Berger, K. W., Martin, J., and Sataloff, R. (1970). The effect of visual distractions on speechreading performance. *Teacher of the Deaf, 68,* 384–387.

Binnie, C. A., Montgomery, A. A., & Jackson, P. L. (1974). Auditory and visual contribution to the perception of consonants. *Journal of Speech and Hearing Research, 17,* 619–630.

Bruhn, M. E. (1949). *Mueller-Walle method of lipreading* (7th ed.). Washington, DC: Volta Bureau.

Bunger, A. M. (1952). *Speech reading—Jena method* (2nd rev.). Danville, IL: Interstate Co.

Cornett, O. R. (1967). Cued speech. *American Annals of the Deaf, 112,* 3–13.

Cornett, O. R. (1972). Effects of cued speech upon speechreading. *International Symposium on Speech Communication Ability and Profound Deafness* (pp. 213–230). Washington, DC: A. G. Bell Association.

Costello, M. R. (1964). Individual differences in speechreading. *Report of the Proceedings of the International Congress on Education of the Deaf and of the Forty-first Meeting of the Convention of American Instructors of the Deaf* (pp. 317–321). Washington, DC: U.S. Government Printing Office.

Craig, W. H. (1964). Effects of preschool training on the development of reading and lipreading skills of deaf children. *American Annals of the Deaf, 109,* 280–296.

Deland, F. (1968). *Story of lip reading: Its genesis and development.* Washington, DC: Volta Bureau.

Erber, N. P. (1974). Effects of angle, distance, and illumination on visual reception of speech by profoundly deaf children. *Journal of Speech and Hearing Research, 17*(1), 99–112.

Evans, L. (1965). Psychological factors related to lipreading. *Teacher of the Deaf, 63*, 131–136.

Hull, R. H. (1976). A linguistic approach to the teaching of speechreading: Theoretical and practical concepts. *Journal of the Academy of Rehabilitative Audiology, 9*, 14–19.

Jeffers, J., & Barley, M. (1971). *Speechreading (lipreading)*. Springfield, IL: Charles C. Thomas.

Kinzie, C. E., & Kinzie, R. (1931). *Lip-reading for the deafened adult*. Philadephia; John C. Winston Co.

Kinzie, C. E., & Kinzie, R. (1936). *Lip-reading for children*. Washington, DC: Volta Bureau.

Lowell, E. L. (1960). Research in speechreading: Some relationships to language development and implications for the classroom teacher. *Report of the Proceedings of the Thirty-ninth Meeting of the Convention of American Instructors of the Deaf* (pp. 68–75). Washington, DC: U.S. Government Printing Office.

Moores, D. F. (1978). *Educating the deaf: Psychology, principles, and practices.* Boston: Houghton Mifflin Co.

Morkovin, B. V., & Moore, L. M. (1948). *Life-situation speechreading through the cooperation of senses* (2nd ed.). Los Angeles: University of Southern California Press.

Nitchie, E. H. (1950). *New lessons in lipreading.* Philadelphia: J. B. Lippincott Co.

Olsen, B. D., Alpiner, J. G., Chevrette, W., Glascoe, J., & Metz, M. J. (1972). The Denver scale for assessment of communication function of hearing-impaired adults. In K. W. Berger, *Speechreading, principles and methods* (p. 174). Kent, OH: National Educational Press, Inc.

O'Neill, J. J., & Oyer, H. (1981). *Visual communication for the hard of hearing* (2nd ed.). Englewood Cliffs, NJ: Prentice-Hall.

Popelka, G. R., & Berger, K. W. (1971). Gestures and speech reception. *American Annals of the Deaf, 116*, 434–436.

Sanders, D. A. (1982). *Aural rehabilitation* (2nd ed.). Englewood Cliffs, NJ: Prentice-Hall.

Simmons, A. A. (1959). Factors related to lipreading. *Journal of Speech and Hearing Research, 2*, 340–352.

Vernon, M., & Mindel, E. D. (1971). Psychological and psychiatric aspects of profound hearing loss. In D. E. Rose (Ed.), *Audiological assessment* (pp. 87–132). Englewood Cliffs, NJ: Prentice-Hall.

Woodward, M. F., & Barber, C. G. (1960). Phoneme perception in lipreading. *Journal of Speech and Hearing Research, 3,* 212–222.

Additional Readings

Bower, S. A., & Bower, G. H. (1976). *Asserting yourself, A practical guide for positive change.* Reading, MA: Addison-Wesley.

Butt, D. S., & Chreist, F. M. (1968). A speechreading test for young children. *The Volta Review, 70,* 225–244.

Castle, D. (1977). Telephone training for the deaf. *The Volta Review, 79,* 373–378.

Craig, W. N. (1964). Effects of preschool training on the development of reading and lipreading skills of deaf children. *American Annals of the Deaf, 109,* 280–296.

DiCarlo, L. M., & Kataja, R. (1951). An analysis of the Utley lipreading test. *Journal of Speech and Hearing Disorders, 16,* 226–240.

Erdman, S. A. (1980). The use of assertiveness training in adult aural rehabilitation. *Audiology, An Audio Journal for Continuing Education, 5* (12).

Harrelson, L. M. (1982). Strategies for the hearing impaired. *Hearing Instruments, 33*(10), 9–10.

Jacobs, M. (1979). *Speechreading strategies.* Rochester, NY: National Technical Institute for the Deaf.

Jeffers, J. (1967, November). *A re-evaluation of the Utley lipreading sentence test.* Paper presented at the Forty-third Annual Convention of the American Speech and Hearing Association, Chicago, IL.

Kaplan, H. (1982). The impact of hearing impairment and the need to facilitate adjustment. In R. H. Hull (Ed.), *Rehabilitative audiology* (pp. 69–80). New York: Grune & Stratton.

Kaplan, H. (1982). Facilitating adjustment. In R. H. Hull (Ed.), *Rehabilitative audiology* (pp. 81–97). New York: Grune & Stratton.

Keaster, J. (1955). An inquiry into current concepts of visual speech reception. *Laryngoscope, 65,* 80–84.

Maurer, J. F., & Rupp, R. R. (1979). *Hearing and aging, Tactics for intervention* (pp. 179–221). New York: Grune & Stratton.

McCarthy, P. A., & Alpiner, J. G. (1978). The remediation process. In J. G. Alpiner (Ed.), *Handbook of adult rehabilitative audiology* (pp. 88–120). Baltimore, MD: Williams & Wilkins.

Nithart, T. (1982). Some practical approaches to hearing rehabilitation. *Hearing Instruments, 33*(10), 14–15.

Pappas, J. J., Graham, G. S., & Rolls, C. R. (1982). Psychological problems associated with hearing impairment. *Hearing Instruments, 33*(10), 22–23.

Pollack, M. C. (1979). The remediation process: Psychological and counseling aspects. In J. G. Alpiner (Ed.), *Handbook of adult rehabilitative audiology* (pp. 121–140). Baltimore, MD: Williams & Wilkins.

Rupp, R. R., & Heavenrich, A. Z. (1982). Positive communicative game rules: Part I. *Hearing Instruments, 33*(9), 34.
Part II. *Hearing Instruments, 33*(10), 16–19.
Part III. *Hearing Instruments, 33*(11), 20–22.

Sanders, D. A. (1980). Hearing aid orientation and counseling. In M. C. Pollack (Ed.), *Amplification for the hearing impaired* (2nd ed., pp. 343–392). New York: Grune & Stratton.

Taaffe, G. (1957). A film test of lip reading. *John Tracy Clinic Research Papers* II. Los Angeles: John Tracy Clinic.

Utley, J. (1946). A test of lipreading ability. *Journal of Speech and Hearing Disorders, 11*, 109–116.

Vognsen, S. (Ed.). (1976). *Hearing tactics.*Fredericia, Denmark: National Council of Health Education, The State Hearing Institute.

Index